# Advance Praise for HEALTHWALK

"Carlson and Seiden know how to walk and how to write unapologetically for the sake of walking. They have provided all the facts in a convincing manner for the entire range of walkers, from cardiac patients to Olympic racewalkers. Their gospel in this inspiring book is: Walk!"

—Bob Kitchen,
Former Chair,
Men's & Women's Racewalking,
The Athletics Congress/USA

"*HealthWalk* is a sensible book on how to make your journey through life healthier through walking."

—Rob Sweetgall,
Creative Walking, Inc.

"A giant step toward a better, healthier outlook on life."

—Henry Laskau,
Lifetime President,
Walkers Club of America

# HealthWalk

# HealthWalk

## To Total Wellness for All Ages

Bob Carlson
O.J. Seiden, M.D.

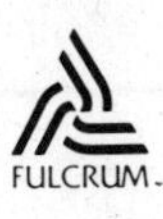


1988

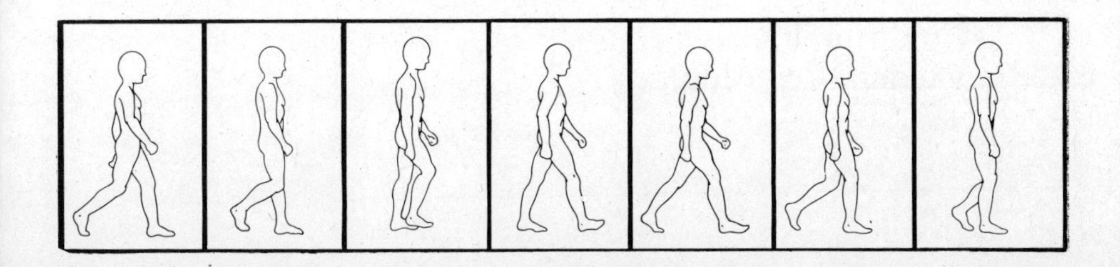

Design by JR Designs



**Library of Congress Cataloging-in-Publication Data**

Carlson, Bob.
HealthWalk/by Bob Carlson and O.J. Seiden.

Bibliography: p.
1. Walking—Health aspects. I. Seiden, Othniel J. II. Title

RA781.65.C37 1988 613.7'1—dc19 88-3531
ISBN 1-55591-028-9 (pbk.)

1 2 3 4 5 6 7 8 9 0

Printed in the United States

Fulcrum, Inc.
Golden, Colorado
1988

Dedicated to my mother, who in her eighties, walks four miles daily and swims 30 minutes three times a week . . . an act we all should follow!

—O.J. Seiden, M.D.

To my mother, Augustine, who at 93 years of age has provided the facilities and encouragement necessary to do my writing, and to my five children, Tina, Bob, Doug, Glenn and Jim, for their moral support in all my endeavors.

—Bob Carlson

# Contents

# FOREWORD

Lifestyle recipes for ways to achieve good health abound. In this book, the authors present us with one that is literally accessible to each of us who is blessed with the too often taken-for-granted ability to walk. It is written for the young who want to preserve their health, as well as for the elderly who want to restore their health. *HealthWalk: To Total Wellness at Any Age* is about shattering our own internalized myths that old age is something to be feared and that there is little that can be done to lessen its impact.

The single most important factor determining our quality of life is our health, and the single most important factor affecting our health is the degree to which we as individuals are willing to take responsibility for our own diets and exercise, no matter what age we are at the present time. We will all inevitably slow down, but the process of aging need not be crippling. Imagine in your future having the good health and energy to enjoy a lifetime of accumulated experience, wisdom and friendships.

Even as we age as individuals, our society is aging. By now, almost everyone is aware that a steadily increasing percentage of the U.S. population is living past 85. Men and women 85 and over constitute the fastest growing age group in the United States. In 1950, half a million people were over 85. By the year 2000, there will be more than five million. Care of the aging will be the number one issue facing our health care systems and it will be competing with other pressing social needs for precious public resources. The least expensive, most fundamental step we can take to prepare for this challenge will be a personal step.

WE MUST TAKE CARE OF OURSELVES.

—Former Governor of Colorado, Richard D. Lamm

# INTRODUCTION

*"That which is used develops. That which is not used wastes away."*
—Hippocrates

---

Isn't it a shame that fitness and its accompanying robust good health cannot be stored? If it could, we could exercise like demons when young, store it up and parcel it out in old age like an IRA account. Unfortunately our bodies don't quite work that way. The way to achieve old-age vigor is to adopt a lifetime aerobic exercise when young and stay with it throughout life. We recommend brisk walking as the perfect program for lifetime health through exercise because of its convenience, lack of injury potential and its myriad other virtues, which are discussed in this book.

It is our purpose here to show you how to live this new lifestyle and have the longest and best-quality future possible. Most important is a program of regular, effective exercise. It is now being demonstrated that the best, the simplest and the most natural form of exercise for us humans is walking—brisk walking. Walking is the cornerstone of this ideal program toward good health and productive longevity. Add to that some common-sense rules of diet and the elimination of destructive bad habits, and you should be able to look forward to a longer future with confidence and excitement.

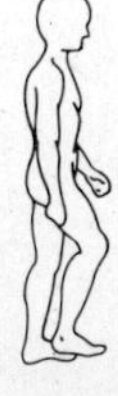

Truly, aging is a natural part of life, but there are two forms of aging: our chronological clock, which we cannot do a thing about, and our biological clock, over which we have great control and which is all-important to our future. In recent years our life expectancies have increased substantially. There is, thankfully, some lengthening taking place in the final years. Medical science has recognized several aspects of our changing lifestyles that have contributed to this phenomenon. Of the utmost importance is that these lifestyle variables not only increase the years we have to live but also improve the quality of life in those added years.

We must take charge of our own destinies and not tempt fate by embracing poor lifestyle habits. We are now experiencing many self-imposed diseases and disabilities, such as heart disease, cancer, hypertension, stroke, chronic respiratory diseases—the major killers and maimers in our society today. We say these are self-imposed because we are indeed bringing them on ourselves. In certain other cultures, with different lifestyles, these fatal or debilitating illnesses are rare; in fact, in olden days, they were not the major causes of death in our own country. Fortunately, we are slowly learning how important fitness is, thanks to all the media attention currently given to healthy lifestyles. A revolution of sorts has begun, and more and more people are realizing that healthy diet and exercise are vital to our health and well-being. Even so, too few of our population are adhering to systematic exercise and health programs adequate to be of real and lasting benefit.

We want to make it clear, lest you think we are addressing solely the elderly in this book, that we hope to motivate people of every age to address their futures. It is surprising what a low priority disease prevention and education about lifetime health habits for the youth of our country has had—especially when you consider the ramifications of this shortsightedness.

## Walking for Children

In *HealthWalk* we are aiding a remarkable gentleman, Rob Sweetgall, in promoting his program designed to teach the youth of America the benefits and joys of lifetime personal fitness through aerobic walking.

Rob left a highly paid job as a chemical engineer for DuPont in 1981 to establish his Foundation for Cardiovascular Fitness and Creative Walking (407-S White Clay Center, Newark, DE 19711). Motivated by the fact that his own family had been devastated by deaths from cardiovascular disease in a short period of time, he now devotes himself to informing others of the vital need to remain active for life.

In 1984–85, to spread the word, Rob trekked solo carrying only a four-pound fanny pack for support, through all 50 states in 50 weeks, covering 11,208 miles. The University of Massachusetts Medical School flew him back to their facility for extensive testing each six weeks to find out what happens to a human body averaging 31 miles of walking every day for a year. Every calorie eaten and all other aspects of what he did every day were meticulously recorded on computers. It became the most involved study of any one person's physiology in history. Rob enjoyed a trip which some might consider the ultimate in self-torture and agony—and he finished in better health than when he started

The whole trip was designed around the scheduling of school assemblies in each state along the designated route. He lectured to around 200 groups of children and administrators during his sojourn. As a result, he developed a new concept of physical education called Walking Wellness, for elementary schoolchildren and teachers. A lifetime fitness manual is provided to help each child keep track of his/her progress in aerobic fitness through the year. Homework assignments and workshops, numbering 16 half-hour sessions per year, cover the major aspects of personal fitness and health. During each lesson, students walk, talk, write, read, reason, calculate, plan, analyze, cooperate and discover. Half the course is physical walking exercise, and the other half is "walking for the mind." No workshop is complete without the homework; the principles of healthy lifestyle are thus put firmly into the students' minds. This concept addresses each student's needs and encourages *all* students (not just the star athletes as in the conventional systems), regardless of ability. Each student competes only with himself or herself as personal improvements are noted.

Initiating and engraving preventive ideas deeply into

students' minds at an early age can have a huge impact on health care in the United States in the future years. Our youth are our future.

An interesting fact of our life is that in 1985 there were 17.1 million women over the age of 65 in the USA and only 11.4 million males. This puts two burdens on the shoulders of our female population: To keep themselves fit, healthy and active so as to survive a probable widowhood, and also to try to keep their husbands from being one of those early statistics. Much can be done to keep male partners alive for many more years than the present American lifestyle tends to allow.

Dr. Seiden started walking to keep a friend company after the friend had a triple-bypass operation. His cardiologist had wisely demanded that he get off his duff and change from the sedentary life that caused him to need a bypass, to an active life that could work against further heart problems. Now their wives are walking regularly too. Rarely do they let their men miss a day of workout. Dr. Seiden knows for sure that he would be far more lax in his exercise, nutrition and general health program if it weren't for his wife's efforts and encouragement. This is all worth keeping in mind.

Dr. Seiden quit his medical practice in the middle 1970s to become an author writing mostly on health-related subjects. He also volunteers his time periodically to assist an organization called Doctors to the World, which sends physicians to underdeveloped sectors of the earth, to establish better health practices in those needy places. Dr. Seiden would dearly love to see the entire populace embrace his own lifestyle habits, of which endurance walking is the cornerstone. His best effort is 78 miles—a triple marathon—in about 18 hours.

Bob Carlson is a veteran of the famed 10th Mountain Division of World War II and a former architect, who gave up his profession (also in the mid-1970s) to devote his life to health promotion and physical fitness. He started as a marathon runner in 1967, but since 1982 has gravitated to walking, especially racewalking, as a far more sensible form of staying in excellent shape. Bob has won many racewalking regional championships and a national one in his 60–64 age group, normally doing the 5 kilometer distance in 29 to 30 minutes. He has done extensive writing and teaching on the benefits of walking as the best exercise for the most people. He is the founder of Colorado's Front Range Walkers Club.

It is our firm belief that if you follow our advice, you can be middle-aged in a physiological and psychological sense far into your later years (80s, 90s and even 100s) and that you can truly "healthwalk" to total wellness.

## CHAPTER 1

# CAN I REALLY INCREASE MY PRODUCTIVE LIFE SPAN?

*"A scientific breakthrough of major significance has been the recognition that many problems long attributed to aging are, in fact, infirmities that could be avoided if people would only be more active. Some of those dreaded infirmities include shortness of breath, slowed reflexes, loss of muscle strength, senility, stiffness of the joints, and soft bones."*

—C. Carson Conrad,
President's Council on Physical Fitness and Sports

---

You bet! There is a growing mass of evidence that says you can. Dr. Ernest Jokl, renowned researcher and authority on aging at the University of Kentucky, has stated: "There is little doubt that proper physical activity as a way of life can significantly delay the aging process." We contend that walking, when done properly and regularly, can completely fill that activity requirement. Walking is the safest, most natural and best aerobic, full-body and cardiovascular exercise available to us. Every indicator we have seen points to this fact:You can walk away from infirmity and old age!

True, old age is not defined in terms of the number of birthdays you've had but in how you act, think and feel—how you function physically and mentally. Although the effects of aging cannot be completely eliminated, they can be slowed and, in part, be reversed to a remarkable degree. The heart and lungs absolutely depend on exercise to supply the body with the real staff of life—oxygen. The only way to develop and maintain a really efficient oxygen transport system in your body is through aerobic exercise.

Aerobic means "with air" and refers to an activity that can

be sustained without your getting breathless—as opposed to anaerobic, which creates an oxygen debt and its resulting breathlessness. Aerobic exercise, as opposed to anaerobic exercise, utilizes maximum oxygen. It works the heart and lungs for longer periods at a time than anaerobics. Anaerobics tend to work muscles against resistance for short spurts of time and uses a minimum amount of oxygen.

As this book will make you realize, a vigorous walking program is by far the most efficient and effective aerobic program that you can have. A vigorous walking program can actually make a heart so strong that it will need to beat only half as fast as an unconditioned heart. People have lowered heart rates of 90 down to 45 or 50. Think what that means! The heart gets twice as much rest between beats because it is so strong and efficient. Exercised lungs that are not contaminated by tars, carcinogens and the harmful chemicals deposited there by smoking tobacco or dope also become much more efficient and can process much more vital oxygen in the bloodstream.

Understand that we are not saying we want to add decrepit years on to the tail end of a decrepit life span. WHAT WE WANT YOU TO DO IS EXTEND THE EXCITING, PRODUCTIVE, MIDDLE YEARS OF YOUR LIFE.

## There Is a Fountain of Youth

Ever since Ponce de Leon sought the fountain of youth hundreds of years ago there have been numerous searches for this elusive goal. It has finally been found. Not by a swashbuckling explorer but by travelers to strange, remote places—gerontologists and volunteer physicians to underdeveloped areas of our world. It was on one of these volunteer medical missions to a remote area in Ecuador, high in the Andes Mountains that Dr. Seiden discovered a way of life that produces extremely healthy old people who are productive and happy in their late 80s, through their 90s and into their early 100s.

Studies from the Hunzas in Northern Pakistan, the Abkhasians in the Caucasus Mountains of Russia, and the Andes in Vilcabamba, Ecuador, where Dr. Seiden observed firsthand, show an inordinate number of persons who have achieved extraordinary longevity and vigorous health. In these places elderly people have had the following characteristics in common:

1. They engage in many hours of physical exertion daily, walking up and down hills and often carrying substantial loads.
2. Their diets are low in animal fats, cholesterol and salt, while high in fiber and vegetable carbohydrates.
3. They do not destroy their bodies with smoking or other harmful chemical abuse.

These people are generally slender, well-muscled, vigorous and youthful in appearance. High blood pressure and cardiovascular disease is virtually unknown. The incidence of cancer is far lower than in our culture. Age is revered by the young in these areas, and the elderly look forward to active life spans of over one hundred years. Heredity is only a part of these peoples' extraordinary life spans; the daily vigorous activity is the biggest factor.

If we could learn from them and adapt our own lifestyles to include some of their good habits, we too can live out our lives to their full potential—not only in longevity but also in activity, productivity and pleasure.

## We've Become a Wheel/Chair Society

Our typical American lifestyles often discourage us from reaching our life potentials. We are provided with a myriad of inventions that allow us to lead a completely sedentary existence, devoid of even a minimum of exercise. In truth we have become a sedentary society—a "wheel/chair society" in which we spend most minutes of the day either riding motorized wheels or sitting in chairs. Staying on this course will only hasten confinement to real wheelchairs in later life.

According to Dr. Fred Schwartz, director of the American Medical Association committee on aging, "Many of the so-called infirmities of old age stem directly from lack of conditioning. Great numbers of people settle into a sedentary life after leaving high school or college. In these circumstances, it is easy to understand why the physical horizons have become cramped and why hands shake and why the gait becomes uncertain and tottery."

From age 30 the average person in our modern society experiences a gradual lowering of functional capacity:

1. Lungs and heart become less efficient at a rate of about 1 percent in cardiac output per year. This can be reversed or avoided.
2. Joints become inflexible, arthritis is common and bones become fragile as calcium and other minerals are lost. These deteriorating events are also avoidable and, to a degree, reversible.
3. Strength declines along with the motivation to exercise and venture out to seek new achievements. This is possibly the most avoidable and reversible of all our aging processes.
4. Tumors seem to appear at random in bones, breasts, skin and vital organs. Our thymus gland (an organ instrumental in the immune system) shrinks and withers, as do other vital organs, and our immune system weakens. We become more susceptible to disease. We are discovering that this is not all due to heredity. Our habits and lifestyles, indeed, have much to do with how rapidly these biologic changes take place and how rapidly we succumb to these changes.
5. After the age of 50, we lose about 3/4 inch in stature per decade; we also have less shoulder width, chest depth and muscular tone and flexibility. Diet and exercise can inhibit this process by 90 percent or more.
6. We lose coordination because of decreased motor response. This is due not to lost talent but because of disuse atrophy, and is thus reversible.
7. We heal slowly from trauma. Activity that improves circulation and diet that effects cell regeneration can accelerate the healing process in elderly people—even to the point where they can heal faster than many younger individuals who have let themselves become sedentary and negligent of their health.
8. Although we tend to start losing weight after the age of 50, it is mainly lean muscle mass we lose and so, actually, we end up with a greater percentage of fatty tissue.
9. If you are, God forbid, a smoker or a heavy alcohol or drug user, almost all of the above aging signs and symptoms

will be accelerated. Have you ever noticed that many heavy smokers experience a wrinkling of their skin much earlier in life than their non-smoking peers? They can appear to be older than their chronological age, and their performance in the activities of life usually follows in the same vein.

If you do not take action and combat these effects of aging, you are apt to end up so frail and weakened that you will eventually succumb to ailments that a more vigorous you could easily withstand. Your arteries will harden, your brain will become less oxygenated and senility may set in. You will become more susceptible to stroke, heart disease, diabetes, blindness, deafness and a multitude of other diseases. This decline in physical and mental functions has always been termed the "normal effects of aging." But all the signs and symptoms listed above are avoidable and/or reversible. We will prove to you in this book that "normal" in this case is not normal after all. It has become "normal" because we have let it become "our norm" in present-day society. It is, in truth, sub-normal.

## Age Has Little to Do with Time

Sadly, old age begins long before chronological middle age for many who are not young at heart. Someone who has enjoyed a healthy lifestyle and has been active throughout life can be younger physiologically and psychologically at 70 than a person of 40 with destructive habits.

Clive Davies of Oregon, in his early 70s, ran 26-mile marathons in about three hours. Can you? Fortunately, you don't need to. You can just walk to stay ahead of old age. But can you walk four miles in one hour? If you can, you are doing very well. If you can't, make that your goal for six months from now. From NOW, not tomorrow! The first destructive habit you must break is putting off to another day what is good for you. Your future health and longevity must become a top priority. It's worth postponing a few things now to give yourself time for good health; you'll have plenty of time for them later when you live longer—longer and more productively.

A law of aging says that any function, skill or tissue that is not continuously used throughout life inevitably will be lost gradually. How often have you seen a vigorous individual retire, then in just a few years lose all vigor and the will to go on? He seems to be on a precipitous decline to a premature grave. On the other hand, an individual who retires and continues to be active, seeking new goals both physically and mentally, seems to thrive, grows in vigor, actually even seems to get younger than before. The difference is attitude. One sees retirement as an end; the other looks forward to it as a beginning, with exciting new challenges and adventures.

Regular use of our physical and mental abilities results in retention of those functions. We all know that muscles that go unused deteriorate, atrophy. (Most of us remember what happens to arms or legs that have been immobilized in plaster casts for several weeks.) The same goes for our mental abilities. What is more important is that unused muscles can be reactivated and can regain their strength, tone and function. So can our brains be revived. The old adage: "You can't teach an old dog new tricks" is a myth. An old mind can learn and develop new knowledge and talents. We can, if we want to and are truly motivated, be middle-aged in our 70s and 80s, instead of being senile, disease-ridden and immobile shells of our former selves.

## Walking Can Restore Mobility

The main reason that many elderly people cannot walk is that they have lost mobility of their hips, knees, ankles and backs. A lot of walking throughout life prevents this problem. If limitation of motion has already begun, the obvious antidote to the condition is to start walking now to counteract further deterioration. In surprisingly little time those joints will limber up, tendons will stretch, muscles will strengthen, balance and grace will return and walking will become easier and pleasurable. The old rocking chair will have to wait.

Dr. Joan Slavin, nutritionist at the University of Minnesota, says that although osteoporosis is considered to be a disease of aging, it can be counteracted by weight-bearing exercise, which maintains bone density and aids in calcium absorption. Numerous experiments have shown that bones have more calcium and are much stronger in elderly exercisers than in their sedentary counterparts. A broken hip can literally be a death sentence to a frail, inactive old person because that person doesn't have the vitality necessary to aid in the healing process. There is too little calcium in his brittle, osteoporotic bones. The active exerciser's bones, on the other hand, can resist breakage to a far greater degree. And even if the bones are broken, they can heal.

## Your Heart Is a Muscle That Needs Exercise

Once walking can be instituted on a regular and vigorous basis, longevity can be expected to increase. The heart is just a muscle. Like other muscles, if it isn't challenged and exercised vigorously, it too tends to weaken and wither. It loses its circulation, and when an emergency arises, it fails. As with any other muscle of the body, exercise strengthens the heart, increases its circulation, and gives it the reserve it needs when called upon to perform in a crisis. That adds up to a longer, more productive life.

## Oxygen—Life's Vital Force

People have been known to last around two months without food before starving to death. A person may last a week without food and water. But without oxygen, brain damage and ensuing death can occur in as quickly as four minutes. Doesn't that make breathing our most important bodily function? The fact is that the more of it we do and the more deeply we breathe, the better it is for our health—mental and physical. Oxygen is the vital fuel of the muscles and the brain. It is our staff of life. The yogis of the Far East have understood the principles of deep breathing and its beneficial effects for many centuries. It is an integral part of their meditation techniques.

Exercise works its magic in rejuvenating powers not by making us hurt, but by making us breathe deeply—a process which oxygenates all of the cells of our bodies. Through aerobic exercise our hearts and lungs remain strong enough throughout life to supply a similar amount of oxygen as our bodies processed when young. Some people who are chronologically old can maintain breathing capacities equal to people 40 years younger. In one experiment, exercise physiologists found that a group of previously unconditioned men and women from 60 to 83 years of age were able to increase their breathing capacities by an average of almost 30 percent in a year's time by doing light calisthenics and walking consistently several times per week. According to physiologists, those gains in aerobic capacity compared very favorably to what might have been expected from people much younger.

## Take a Deep Breath

Let's look at some specifics of the breathing process. The respiratory muscles of the diaphragm and the intercostals (ribs) create a vacuum in the lungs by expanding them in size. The more strenuous the exercise, the more the lungs expand and the more oxygen is drawn in to the body system for its use. There are actually three types of breathing, all of them incomplete unless aided by aerobic exercise.

1. Abdominal (or belly) breathing, which results from lowering the diaphragm and extending the abdomen.
2. Intercostal breathing in the middle of the chest is produced by the contraction of the intercostal muscles between the ribs.
3. The very tops of the lungs are ventilated by the muscular elevation of the collar bones during an inhalation, called clavicular breathing.

All of these individual patterns aid in the breathing process, but they are incomplete in themselves, and, unless you have trained like a yogi, only partially fill the lungs with air. The yogis concentrate on each of these breathing patterns, starting with the abdominal in an attempt to fill the lower lobes completely, then fill the middle lungs, and finally raise the shoulders to fill the upper lobes.

The yogis claim that since the vitality of the lungs is greatly improved by deep breathing, the lining of the lungs is better able to resist the invasion of bacteria and viruses. As a result, the incidence of flu, colds and pneumonia is dramatically reduced. In addition, the quality of the blood is greatly improved by added oxygenation. Consequently all the body functions—the organs and the muscles—benefit in a big way. Also, the up and down movement of the diaphragm massages the stomach and other organs of digestion, causing food to be propelled along faster, and making additional blood available to aid in the digestion process.

All these benefits of deep breathing have been shown to be true over the centuries, but we don't have to study and meditate to get the benefits. All we have to do is get out and walk briskly, breathe deeply, and get in much better shape than if we just sat around deep breathing, yogi-like. We can thus expand our capillary network, exercise the heart muscle, stimulate the enzyme system and burn calories—all of which require oxygen—and supply this oxygen by walking fast and breathing deeply.

The great Australian coach, Percy Cerutty, taught his athletes to pull their shoulders up and raise their arms periodically while running in order to get the lungs completely full to the top of the lobes. He understood that this action added to their aerobic power, and thus their strength and endurance. Experiment to find your ideal breathing pattern and stick with it until it becomes automatic. You will experience all the benefits that complete oxygenation of the blood can bestow on you.

## Walking Helps Circulation

To maintain a strong heart and body, the young should begin early to exercise daily. The elderly also must exercise daily, and with increasing vigor, or else suffer the immobility and infirmities normally associated with old age. The same can be said about our mental abilities as our physical prowess. Inactivity leads to senility—activity keeps us mentally fit. Senility has been associated with hardening of the arteries and poor circulation to the brain.

Poor circulation is also the reason most elderly people don't like cold weather. The answer, again, is regular and vigorous exercise. If you have good circulation, cold weather won't be nearly the threat it would be otherwise.

The elderly need not be total victims of their circulatory system. They have considerable control of their fate. The earlier they take control, the greater that control will be.

## Walking Works Against Aging

The characteristics that normally occur in advancing age for Americans are progressive increase in body fat; loss of muscle mass, tone and strength; decline in physical and mental vigor; increase in triglycerides and cholesterol; increased incidence of elevated blood pressure, heart disease and cancer. These changes are so common in our country that normal standards have been lowered, and many physicians now consider these low standards as "normal" for our elderly. These sub-normal "norms" are just the opposite from those of the people we mentioned earlier from Ecuador, the Caucasus and the Hunzas of Northern Pakistan.

Perhaps genetics has something to do with our accelerated rate of aging compared to those folks who live to be over 100, but lifestyle can make a dramatic change in the way we age. Proper diet, increased exercise rather than decreased activity, and the elimination of a few bad habits can make the difference between experiencing a longer more productive life or a steady deterioration both mentally and physically.

The average human life span has been dramatically increased through the past two decades. In ancient Greece the average life span was only 18 years. In Caesar's time it was up to 22. It reached 35 when the settlers started to arrive in America, and it reached 49 at the turn of the 19th century. At the present time in the United States, the average male can look forward to 73 and females to 78.

But in the past decade that average has been raised at the elderly end. In the 1930s a man looked forward to the ripe old age of 60 as his goal. After World War II, 65 was considered to be a good and full life. Today if a man dies at 65 we say, "What a shame he died so young." We are now used to seeing people who take care of themselves enjoy life to its fullest at that age. We think in terms of late 70s and 80s. We no longer want to retire at 65. Awareness of the benefits of personal lifestyle improvement and medical science are allowing us longer and more productive lives. However, not enough people are adhering to the correct lifestyle principles. If you are one of them, take heed.

The earlier in life you begin your walking program, the greater longevity and productivity you can expect. Even if you are beginning in your later years, you will still be rewarded with remarkable results. But you must begin NOW.

Doubts?

Just read on . . .

CHAPTER 2

# EXERCISE DOESN'T NEED TO BE STRENUOUS

*"Most of the men I have met between the ages of 40 and 70 could make themselves feel years younger by taking to the open road and—barring hearts that are too far gone to be salvaged—could be assured of longer and happier lives. . . . As for the younger men, sometimes in watching the mad pace of modern life, I wonder if they are not more in need of hikes than their grandfathers. Walking would teach them the quality that youngsters find so hard to learn—patience. It would give them proof that the race is not always to the swift."*

—Edward Payson Weston,
Premier U.S. walker of the 19th century

---

It was thought until recent years that the only way to get into very good shape was to struggle through tough workouts, and that "no pain, no gain" was the rule for success. If you strive to be an Olympic champion, or even just the best in your age group, this may be true. But for most of us it is not.

Let's look into this idea of fitness by going clear back into prehistory to our ancestor the caveman. What sort of shape do you suppose he was in? Part of the logic behind our fitness-seeking is that it relates to a condition that has evolved from the caveman: the survival instinct. If the cavemen were in the marvelous shape and as strong as the anthropologists think, they would probably be very adept in today's exercise activities requiring strength and endurance. Every bit of the work our prehistoric forebears did to survive was done manually, with no mechanical help. Undoubtedly, their entire day was one constant endurance effort, having to walk everywhere they went, carrying loads in their arms and hands or on their backs and shoulders. Our bodies were designed for this type of living initially, and they are still—ALMOST. In just the last century we have strayed away from endurance exercise with all our labor-saving devices. We thus have brought upon ourselves ailments such as heart disease, lung cancer, hypertension, stroke and other environmentally and self-induced cancers and illnesses that have in the past been far rarer. We have replaced the infectious diseases, now easily curable, that plagued man throughout history with self-inflicted ones caused by terrible lifestyle habits, including sedentariness, poor nutrition and chemical abuse of many kinds.

The caveman's lifestyle was not too far removed from that of the modern-day people in the remote areas of Northern Pakistan, Ecuador, the Caucasus Mountains of Russia and other primitive societies of the world. We have already told you that in these areas an inordinate number of people live to remarkable and vigorous old age. We are not saying that you need to return to a primitive lifestyle and give up all your modern pleasures and possessions, but we are recommending that you keep the best of both worlds. Enjoy your modern life but take with it what modern science is now rediscovering as the key to the real productive longevity we were meant to achieve.

We're writing about endurance and not sprint training or exercise that requires quick bursts of energy. We're writing about the type of fitness that walks of relatively low intensity, but of long duration, can bring. Endurance and not lightning speed is the key to the type of aerobic fitness that is the most important for our health and well-being. We're writing about activities that are done consistently almost every day and that allow us to keep our strength and agility throughout life.

Did the caveman run? Surely, for short distances, to catch some animal, to flee another. But most of his time was spent walking and tracking his prey. The women and children spent their time gathering provisions. Running was unnecessary most of the time. Authorities say that they never really pushed themselves. They didn't need to. They got a steady dose of milder exercise all day, every day, which was enough to keep them in top shape until the time either mishap, infection or old age ended their stay on earth. We're willing to bet that they weren't afflicted with the hamstring pulls and the knee injuries that runners suffer from today.

If running or weight training or aerobics and calisthenics are not your style, then take a lesson from your ancestor the caveman and walk your way to fitness. It's the natural way to get into shape.

## Walking Is Ideal Exercise for the Expectant Mother

A special word should be said about pregnancy. Walking is an ideal workout program for an expectant mother. It helps circulation for both the mother and the fetus, and it keeps the weight under control. It strengthens the pelvic muscles important for delivery, aids the circulation for her and the unborn fetus, and will make her labor easier. After the baby is born, walking should be continued, building up gradually and carrying the little rascal along if weather permits. This will be beneficial both for you and your child. Your health advisor should be supportive of the right intensity of exercise to keep the body toned.

## Mild Exercise Is Good Medicine

We Americans are often too impatient. We want immediate results. There is the belief that the harder the training, the quicker we will get into shape—but most often the reverse is true. Overtraining is the cause of great discouragement and frustration, causing strained and sore muscles, tired feet and a generally "washed-out feeling." Naturally we do not look forward to these less-than-delightful symptoms. Only the physically gifted can stand the PTA method of training (Pain, Torture and Agony).

The main reason that brisk walking has the lowest dropout rate of all exercises regularly practiced by Americans is that going out for a walk is not nearly as intimidating or as hard on the body as going out for a jog or run. And you can't beat the convenience factor, since we all walk some place for some distance every day, whether we want to or not. All we need to do to get into fine shape is to increase the intensity and time period of the exercise.

In a study by Dr. D. Willem Erkelens, published in the *Journal of the American Medical Association*, 83 heart-attack patients were put on a mild exercise program for 45 minutes per day three days per week. The program was consistent walking or slow jogging and light calisthenics; it continued for six months. After this period the intensity of the exercise increased only slightly, but the HDL cholesterol (High Density Lipids, the good kind) had increased by an average of 12 percent. The conclusion was that "the amount of exercise for this noteworthy improvement in the blood lipids was not very great." California endocrinologist Dan Streja, M.D., reinforced this idea when he stated: "To favorably alter cholesterol, to lower blood sugar, insulin and triglyceride levels, and to lose weight, walking will do it. Metabolically speaking, walking is as good as running."

In another experiment at the San Diego State College Exercise Laboratory, 23 hypertensive men were put on a regimen of less than strenuous exercise consisting of 15 minutes of warm-up calisthenics plus a half hour of walking or slow jogging twice a week. After six months their mean blood pressure had fallen from 159/105 to 146/93—close to normal range.

Yet another study was conducted by Dr. George V. Mann and colleagues of the Vanderbilt School of Medicine, in order to find a feasible system of supervised exercise that they could measure against the effects on heart disease risk factors. The 105 men studied included professionals, blue-collar and white-collar workers, and a few laborers. They were able to attend sessions for an hour either before or after work. There was always a trained leader present, and the exercise consisted of warm-up calisthenics followed by alternate walking and jogging. They were placed into three groups according to their initial fitness, and as they improved they were upgraded into higher levels. The program lasted six months and 76 percent of the participants stuck with it for the entire period; 96 percent of the 105 said that they would do it again and complete it if they had the chance. The end result was that there was a big improvement in feelings of well-being and fitness, there was a significant decrease in body fat without dietary restrictions, blood lipid profiles improved and blood pressures fell significantly. In analyzing the results, Dr. Mann was able to conclude that only three fairly non-strenuous sessions per week are needed to produce measurable benefits and better health. We still, however, recommend more frequent exercise for best results.

## Low-Intensity Exercise Is Beneficial

Walking is as good as running in a metabolic sense. Metabolics (the ability of the body to convert food to energy) are all you really need to think about unless you're attempting to be a star athlete. High-intensity exercise does increase the HDL level more than low-intensity exercise, but only by a small amount. We contend that this small difference is not worth the effort or the strain on the body, particularly if this is a deterrent to exercising. You will not get any benefits from exercise not done, hence you should walk.

Aerobic exercise for your circulation and respiration is meant to work your heart harder than usual—but the critical question is: How much harder? If you do too little, you improve at a frustratingly slow rate. As we have said, too much is even more frustrating. The best way to monitor yourself to make sure that you do the proper amount is to stay around your ideal pulse rate, the definition of which is in Chapter 6, "Little Goals—Bigger Goals." With a little practice you can tell without even stopping when you are in your training zone. A good rule is that if you can't talk while you are exercising, you are going at it too hard.

There are plenty of beneficial levels in between very hard exercise and no exercise at all. Those millions of years of evolution have trained us to become not sprinters, or long-distance cyclists, or weight lifters, or anything other than walkers—brisk hour-long walkers. Almost all of us can be good at it—so good in fact that there is misplaced but widespread doubt as to its benefits, because it seems far too easy. Therein lies the beauty of the exercise—we can get into very good shape doing something that is second-nature to us, very easy to do and very pleasurable as well.

# CHAPTER 3

# WHY IS WALKING THE BEST EXERCISE?

*"A vigorous five-mile walk will do more good for an unhappy but otherwise healthy adult than all the medicine and psychology in the world."*

—Paul Dudley White, M.D.,
Former dean of American cardiologists

---

People will ask you: "Why walk?" Here is the ammunition to defend your new sport and fitness activity.

It's often hard to convince most people that walking is a superior exercise because nearly everyone does it. We take the activity for granted and are therefore blind to its benefits. But consider its advantages:

1. Walking is the best exercise at any age. Of all exercises it is the safest and least traumatic to your body. You were designed to walk for great distances and sometimes at remarkable speeds. This was true even back in the day of the caveman when people ran only for the hunt and in emergencies. The human body was not made to withstand the punishment of long and continuous running and jogging—lifting the weight completely off the ground and landing on a bent leg with each jarring step.

2. Walking exercises the entire body and mind. It utilizes the upper body more than running and the legs far more than swimming. In a vigorous and brisk walk, there is virtually no muscle system in your body at rest. And as you will learn later,

it stimulates mental and creative activity better than any other aerobic exercise.

3. You will probably burn more calories, exercise your heart, lungs and circulation better, lose more weight, and develop your body and mind better than you could in any other activity that is so convenient and easy to do.

4. Your walking program will give you the best cardiovascular/cardiopulmonary workout you can get, and with the greatest margin of safety.

5. In addition, walking will lower your blood pressure, help reduce your stress and triglyceride levels, and can take off one pound a week with just a minor alteration of your diet.

6. Walking is a family sport, one of the few that all ages can partake in equally and together. It can be done by virtually anyone, anytime, anywhere. More than 40 percent of the American public will tell you that walking is their main source of exercise—and Americans are relative newcomers to walking as a fitness activity.

7. Your continuing self-improvement through regular walking will be all that you will need to keep you moving toward your goals.

8. If competition is what you want, see Chapter 8. Race-walking is an Olympic event of rapidly growing interest. Numerous race-walking competitions are held almost any weekend during spring, summer and fall in cities all over the USA and other parts of the world. Competition is stiff in all age groups, over courses from one mile to five, 10, 15, 20, 30 and 50 kilometers. In how many other sports can you compete into your 80s or older?

## Walk, Don't Run?

Well, these are mighty big claims. Let's look at some of the evidence that backs them up.

Calories burned are dependent completely on energy spent. Energy spent is dependent on moving mass (body weight) through distance. In other words, the number of calories your body burns and the energy it expends has to do mainly with how far you move. Speed has a surprisingly small effect on energy used and calories burned if you are moving

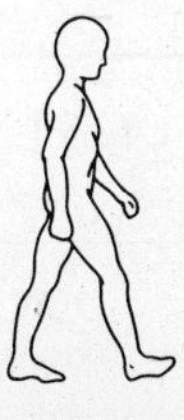

faster than a stroll. This means, if you run or jog a mile, you'll burn just a few more calories than if you walk that same mile at a reasonable speed of say three or four mph. But, beware, if you walk too slowly, such as at two mph, your movement is so efficient that far fewer calories are expended.

So far, all things are equal. The walker is no better off than the jogger or runner. But what of the aerobic value of the exercises? Which will do the cardiovascular system the most good? Here is where we start to see a difference.

The most recent studies in sports medicine are showing that for a person to get cardiovascular aerobic benefit, he must burn off at least 2,000 calories a week at a pace that will keep the pulse steadily above a minimum figure for that person's age. That figure will fall between 110 to 170 pulse beats per minute for most of us, depending on our age. For maximum benefit to your heart and lungs, you must maintain your ideal pulse rate for 45 minutes to an hour. (On page 47 is a simple formula with which to calculate your ideal pulse rate.) Very few runners or joggers can or will do that. The average jogger runs less than 20 minutes three days a week. If in those 20 minutes they can jog three miles (which few can), they would be burning about 300 calories, which is far short of the 2,000-calorie requirement. At five times per week the jogger would burn 1,500 calories, still 500 short, and still be nowhere near the 45-minute workout required to get maximum aerobic benefit. A walker, on the other hand, can quite easily walk a 15-minute-mile speed for an hour (after a few weeks of conditioning) or for four miles. That will burn off 400 calories—or 2,000 calories in just five days, 2,800 in seven days (well over the minimum)—and means you maintain the pulse rate not just for 45 minutes but for a full 60. And in doing this type of workout you are subjecting yourself to far less trauma and chance for injury.

Running has one of the highest incidences of ankle, knee, hip and back injuries of any sport. Just pick up any running magazine and you will find it half full of articles and letters to the editor about how to avoid self-imposed injuries or how to recover as soon as possible.

To develop a running program that would be as effective as a one-hour walk a day would likely require months of conditioning, Herculean will power and many painful hours of rehabilitation, unless you are among the 20 to 25 percent who are biomechanically suited for running. It's not likely that you would stick with it for more than a few weeks, and for this program to work it has to be for life. Only walking can be, for most people, for life. The average runner puts at least three times his body weight of impact on his joints and back with each jarring step he takes. For a 150-pounder it means 450 pounds of impact on ankles, knees, hip and lower back. For most of us that spells injury, arthritis, sprains, strains, twists, stress, stress fractures and pain, pain, pain. That means the end of the workout program—and back to the downhill slide.

## How Walking Compares

The great exercise guru, Dr. Kenneth Cooper, who runs the Aerobics Center in Dallas, Texas, has stated: "Of all the aerobic exercises, walking most nearly puts us in a state of equilibrium and is thus the most consistent with current wellness philosophy." He has also stated that walking 10 minutes per mile or faster (for the ambitious ones that can attain this kind of speed) and vigorous cross-country skiing rate at the top of the list of overall aerobic exercises, above swimming, rowing, running and bicycling.

Let's take a look at the various activities that you might consider for your exercise program:

*Swimming:* Very good for the upper body, but not much for the legs. Since it is non-weight bearing, it does nothing to strengthen the skeletal system. A good aerobic sport if you swim at least 45 minutes a day. Requires a fairly long pool to give you maximum benefit. Swimming is an excellent adjunct to a walking program. If possible, swim in addition to walking or on days when you cannot walk for some reason.

*Bicycling:* Most of us let the bicycle do most of the work. If you don't coast and you pedal hard enough to keep your pulse at your ideal level, bicycling is good, but to do that for 45 minutes or longer, you'll have to ride a long, long way—maybe 20 or more miles. Like swimming, it is non-weight bearing. It can also be fairly dangerous and expensive. It provides very good leg exercise, especially for the quadriceps (front of thigh). The stationary bike is better in that you don't tend to coast and will keep up a steady pace. An excellent aerobic adjunct to your walking program for days when you can't walk. But it is tedious—unless you can set up a rack to read this book as you cycle!

*Rowing:* Excellent aerobic exercise, but doing it on a machine is as tedious as stationary bicycling or swimming. If you have a lake to row on, it is one of the best aerobic exercises, but few of us have this luxury. Should be done for 45 minutes at a time. Expensive. Good cross-training for walking.

*Rope jumping:* A very strenuous and strong aerobic workout. For that reason it is extremely difficult to maintain for more than a few minutes. It is hard to recommend this exercise as one that could be maintained long enough to give much aerobic benefit. Pounds on the legs about as much as running. A great deal of coordination is required to do this exercise for long without a lot of interruptions.

*Roller skating:* A very good activity aerobically, and fun, but can be rather dangerous due to the inability to dodge things quickly or brake adequately. Should be done in flat, unobstructed areas while wearing protective elbow and knee pads.

*Court sports:* Racquetball, handball, volleyball and tennis are all fun sports and good exercise as long as they are played hard with people of somewhat equal ability. The fact is that most people do them strictly for fun, and therefore don't put a lot of effort into them. The movement, though sometimes vigorous, is not constant enough and may be classed as "anaerobic" (without oxygen) in nature. They are stop-and-start exercises. The pulse is not maintained at a steady rate as required for aerobic improvement. Pulse rates will vary between 90 and 170, with the the elevated rates being too brief to do any good. These sports are a good adjunct to your walking program, but there is a relatively high risk of minor injuries.

*Team sports:* Softball, flag football, bowling, etc. are all fun, but too much time is spent waiting for something to happen. They are not very good cardiovascular exercises because of their anaerobic nature, and they are fraught with danger of minor to major injuries. Soccer is probably the best team sport aerobically, followed by basketball. Good adjuncts to walking because they are fun and likely to be continued because of their social nature.

*Weight training:* Weight lifting, body building and Nautilus-type workouts are OK for strength building but not for aerobics. Avoid these if you have any tendency toward high blood pressure. They are strictly anaerobic in nature. Do these if you enjoy them, but they are not necessary at all for your walking program.

## Aerobic vs. Anaerobic

Anaerobic exercises are those that utilize muscular activity for short periods of time, as in running the 100-meter dash or running out a hit. It is estimated that the first two to four minutes of any exercise are anaerobic, utilizing energy stored within the muscles themselves. Anaerobic exercises do little for your cardiovascular/cardiopulmonary systems. This does not mean that anaerobics do not burn oxygen; all activity does. But anaerobics usually work muscles against resistance for short spurts at a time and do not exercise the heart and lungs sufficiently. Most of them have a decided strengthening effect, but you don't much hear of people dying from lack of strength. If you want to gain weight or sculpture a physique, mix anaerobic and aerobic workouts for body building and strength training. Walking is a great co-exercise for weight trainers.

Aerobic exercises are those that utilize maximum oxygen. They work the heart and lungs vigorously and steadily for long periods of time. Aerobics tend to increase endurance while they tone and build muscles. You usually burn more calories and storage fat than with anaerobics, and the total amount of work you do during aerobics is usually cumulatively greater.

Walking is an excellent conditioner for any other sport. Any activity that is enjoyable can be pursued as an adjunct to your walking program, but it will not serve as a substitute. Walking is as complete an exercise as you will need to get into and stay in superb shape, and it is for life. But you must do it daily and vigorously, for 45 minutes or more, to get the best results.

## Physiological Benefits

Let's review the advantages that a walking program can bestow upon us:

1. It reduces the likelihood of cardiovascular and cerebrovascular disease by increasing blood flow and size of the blood vessels.
2. It strengthens and tones the major muscles of the body, including the heart. It encourages collateral circulation to the heart muscle, which can dramatically increase your chance of surviving a coronary were it to occur.
3. It slows the heart rate by increasing stroke volume (the volume of blood it pumps with one contraction.)
4. It tends to reduce the height to which arterial pressure rises during exercise and stress, and creates a stabilizing effect on blood pressure.
5. It increases the flexibility of joints and muscles, and reduces aches and pains in the back, neck and other body joints.
6. It increases the oxygen supply to the brain, which improves mental sharpness and increases the potential for creative thought.
7. It circulates more oxygen to all body tissues.
8. It reduces blood-fat (triglyceride) levels.
9. It gradually increases high-density (good) cholesterol and lowers low-density (bad) cholesterol.
10. It tones up the glandular system and increases thyroid gland output.
11. It increases the production of red blood cells by the bone marrow and aids lymphatic circulation and blood circulation in general.
12. It augments the alkaline reserve of the body and improves strength and physical efficiency, which can be significant in an emergency requiring extended effort. It benefits body growth and recovery from trauma.
13. It causes muscles to move vital fluids throughout the body, which lessens the work done by the heart. It improves digestion and elimination of body wastes.
14. It releases the flow of endorphins, which are the body's

own natural tranquilizers, and improves coordination by activating neurotransmitters and training the muscle fibers.

15. It reduces the incidence of minor illnesses, allergies, headaches and abdominal problems.

16. It increases the ability to store and utilize nutrients, which increases endurance.

17. It stimulates the metabolism, and this effect continues burning calories for hours after the cessation of exercise, thereby reducing the likelihood of your getting too fat.

18. It has a hardening and strengthening effect on the bones of the entire skeletal system.

19. It increases respiratory capacity and aerobic power.

20. It reduces insomnia and counteracts fatigue.

21. It tends to retard the aging process and present a more youthful appearance.

22. It greatly improves mental outlook, optimism, morale and self-esteem.

Now go out and take a nice walk. When you come back we'll start you on your first steps and make sure that you go about it correctly for your maximum benefit.

CHAPTER 4

# GETTING STARTED

*"Few men know how to take a walk. The qualifications are endurance, plain clothes, old shoes, an eye for Nature, good humor, vast curiosity, good speech, good silence and nothing too much."*

—Ralph Waldo Emerson

---

Since practically everyone learns to walk sometime between the ages of ten months and two years, you may think that we are a little presumptuous in telling you how to do it. It is true that all we need to do is put one foot in front of the other, move out and let the body's unique structure take over. Nevertheless, between those first steps as an infant that cause a lot of hoopla, and the time when we are too old and crippled to walk but wish we could, walking does not receive the attention it deserves.

Walking seems too easy because we are so good at it. We were designed for it. In walking there is a perfect balance between gravitational force and the momentum of forward motion. It's the most natural exercise for the body. Paradoxically, walking at slow to brisk speeds is less tiring than standing in one place. Do you question that? Just stand up and stay put, at ease if you like, for fifteen minutes. Then go take a walk at any speed between a stroll and a brisk walk. Which one is more tiring?

Each of us has our own individual style of walking; it would be a mistake to try to alter your natural style. Our main purpose is to explain how to maximize your benefits from the exercise. For most people this means a gradual increase in intensity or work load until you have reached the point where a "training effect" is felt. The term "gradual" is the key. In the beginning, you should temper your enthusiasm so that you can progress without strain. The old term "no pain, no gain" has proven false where getting into good shape is concerned.

## Why Should We Walk for Wellness?

Motivation is what will determine your success or failure in this effort. If you are not personally motivated, you will probably not stick with any program for your own betterment. No one can force you to live healthier and longer. You need to want it enough to make even minimal efforts to better yourself. Let's look at a few reasons why a person might want to look to the future and walk to total wellness:

1. I want to live as long as possible to enjoy my family and loved ones.
2. I want my family and loved ones to be able to enjoy me as long as possible, and not have to care for an old person's failing, feeble mind and body.
3. I don't want to leave my spouse a young widow/widower.
4. I want to enjoy a long and active retirement.
5. I love my life, and I want to keep on loving it as long as I can.
6. I don't know how long I'll live, but I want to be the healthiest possible for its duration.
7. I want to see and enjoy my grandchildren, great grandchildren and, God willing, great great grandchildren . . . and I want them to enjoy me.
8. When my time comes I want to be remembered as a vigorous old person who went out having a good time.
9. It hurts me to visit my friends in nursing homes; I surely don't want someone to have to visit me in one.
10. I feel good now and I intend to keep feeling good for as long as I live.

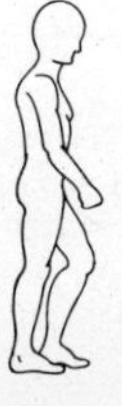

Reasons enough. Chances are you have your own to add to the list. The point is, if you don't do something about it right now, you'll be in worse shape next week, next month, next year—closer to the end of that downhill slide into the hole at the bottom. No matter what your age, now is when you should start your walk back up that hill.

## Take Charge of Your Destiny

If you start to turn your life around today, next year at this time you will be not only just a chronological year older than today, but you'll be trimmer, healthier, better looking, happier, more energetic—more productive than you were, not this year, not last year, but about five years ago. That was our choice, and it is one you too should make today. Turn your act around and start getting physically and psychologically younger as you get chronologically older—before you start losing productive, active, potentially healthy, happy years at about twice the rate of your chronologic aging.

If you follow the program outlined in this book, you'll wrinkle slower, smile longer, laugh harder, feel better, whistle louder, sleep deeper, hug harder, sing better, travel farther, and see and experience more than you ever dreamed possible. Or—you can sit down in the old rocker and deteriorate and doze and ache and wait for the inevitable as life passes you by.

Most of the knowledgeable authorities and researchers in the field of gerontology now agree that the human animal was designed and constructed to last happily for well over a century. The famed British physician Alex Comfort has stated: "It is quite possible that extensions of as much as 10 to 20 percent in useful life span may not be too far in the distant future if the present trends in lifestyle improvement continue at their increasing rates."

At the age of 65 we shouldn't be asking: "Where should we pasture for the next 10 years?" The question we should be asking at that age is: "What shall we do to get the most fun out of the second half of our lives?" The terrible truth is that too many of us are throwing away nearly half of our potential life spans. Too many of us at 70 think it's over. Not so in other parts of the world. Some 70-year-olds are looking forward to

30 and even 40 years' more pleasure. But the first thing you have to do is repair the toll the last few decades have taken. Of course if you are young, you can easily avoid problems by taking charge of your life immediately.

We're assuming that if you're reading this book, you're feeling motivated, so let's get started right now with your new beginning. It is important not to overwhelm you with too many changes at once. We will go about your transformation a stage at a time. Most important now is to get you up off your behind and into exercise. We intend to make it as easy and effective as possible. After you're really into your exercise program, we will shift you to a proper diet gradually, so as to shock your system as little as possible, and then we will go to work on any rotten habits that you might have.

## Walking Is All It Takes

Your new exercise program is based completely on walking. It will start out walking and continue walking. Any other activity will be added only because you want to add it. No other activity is necessary. Walking has it all, can do it all, will do it all. There is no better exercise for you, your body or your mind.

When your body was designed, it was designed for walking. We will teach you to walk so you will obtain the maximum benefit—more than you could benefit from running, jogging, swimming, rope jumping, court sports or any other activity you can think of. In the following chapters you will learn:

- Why walking is by far the best exercise for you at any stage of your life;
- How to get the most out of your walking program;
- What type of walking program is best for you;
- How to set goals realistically;
- How to reach these goals in the most efficient manner.

So now if you are ready for immortality, let's get started. Lay down this book for a half hour and take a walk—an easy walk or stroll. See how far you can get in half an hour and note it. That may be the shortest exercise walk you take for the rest of your life.

Take your walk at your own best pace. Don't force it.

Enjoy it. Look around at the sights. Listen to the sounds. Watch the world pass by at two or three or four miles per hour. Rediscover your neighborhood, or wherever you take those first steps of your new beginnings. Apologies for the cliché, "Today is the first day of the rest of your life." But it really is.

## Walk Tall!

Stand tall with a slight forward lean and walk with an erect posture. Consciously relax your muscles and walk as comfortably as possible. Tight muscles tire very easily, so keep concentrating on looseness of the entire body as you go along. Everyone must experiment to find a natural stride and rhythm. Walk at a good pace, but do not over-stride because if your heel gets too far in front there might be a braking action. Use the arms and shoulders to aid in propulsion. You should be getting the benefits of a full-body, overall exercise. Let your muscles stretch.

Always keep your feet pointed straight ahead, and walk on a real or imaginary straight line for the highest efficiency and the least strain on the leg muscles. If the feet splay either out or in too much, efficiency is lost and strain can result. Don't be afraid to let the hip, lower back and abdominal muscles do their share of the work load. They need toning also.

The more the hips move in a rolling forward and down motion, the less strain there will be on the legs. As your heel strikes the ground, pull it back, pretending the ground is a treadmill, and keep the striding foot on the ground until you feel that your toes are pushing off at the rear of the stride. Ideally your striding foot is on the ground at least two-thirds of the time.

You should land on the outside of the heel and push off with all five toes for the utmost efficiency and power. A 5 percent forward lean from the ankles is ideal to help with your momentum. Do not bend forward at the waist, because it shortens your stride and compromises your breathing power by cramping the lungs. Rotate your hips but don't sway them side to side (looks odd and is not efficient).

Tightness in the hips is why the elderly have trouble walking efficiently. If you feel minor soreness in the shins or hips, don't worry. You are merely using long-neglected muscles; it is only normal to feel a little strain on muscles that have been dormant too long. The more they ache, the more you need this book. If you let your arms dangle at your sides, centrifugal force will push blood to the fingertips and your hands will swell. To eliminate this problem, we recommend that you keep your elbows bent at a 90-degree angle as the arms swing.

Start out slowly on your walks and gradually build up to speed as you go along. The best warm-up exercise for walking is walking slowly. Increase your pace until you feel you are getting a good workout. As we will prove to you throughout this book, you truly can trim down, get rid of that ugly fat, feel much better mentally and physically, and just plain look attractive and healthy. Remember, your health is your true wealth.

Now get up and start walking—life was never intended to be merely a spectator sport. Enjoy yourself. And when you get back in about 30 minutes, start on Chapter 5.

CHAPTER 5

# FIRST STEPS

*"Where the heart is willing, it will find a thousand ways, but where it is unwilling it will find a thousand excuses."*

—Dayak proverb (Borneo)

---

As with any other physical activity, it is best to get into vigorous walking gradually. Walking can be anything from a two-mile stroll to nine-mile-an-hour world-class racewalking. Fifteen kilometers (9.3 miles) has been walked in less than an hour by the world champions, which we can marvel at but needn't be concerned with. We should try, though, to maximize our own performance according to where we start. We must all do the very best we can with the deck of cards that we are dealt by the Creator at birth. If you play those cards poorly you will be missing the true joy of living—vigorous, excellent health. We must all do our best to maximize our own potential, whatever it might be. The walking pace for someone 80 years old varies greatly from that of a youthful athlete, yet both can get the same relative benefit from the exercise, and the 80-year-old has the greater potential for improvement.

## Warm Up to Walking by Walking

Since virtually all of us walk to some degree already, we can get into this vigorous activity rapidly. We do not recommend a long tedious pre-walk warm-up. Actually the best warm-up for walking is walking—slowly at first, then building up gradual intensity to your best aerobic pace as you go along. Walking is in fact the best warm-up for any aerobic or anaerobic activity. Even if you are determined to be a good runner, walk an increasingly rapid half mile first, then proceed into a slow and increasingly faster jog or run.

Nothing warms up cold muscles better than a brisk walk. People have injured themselves during warm-up stretches. It is preferable to warm up with slow walking and then do your stretches as a cool-down when your muscles are well suffused with blood and oxygen. Stretching exercises as a cool-down will help prevent post-workout aches, pains and stiffness, and you will be eager to repeat the exercise the next day.

## Build from What You Can Do Today

If you took that first half-hour walk we recommended at the end of Chapter 4, we can begin with that as our baseline ability. If you didn't do it then, put the book down now and go out for a comfortable 30-minute walk at a pace you can tolerate without getting breathless. Note how far you walked. That will be your baseline. Mark it in a copy of the log that is on page 181–183.

How far did you go? How do you figure how far and how fast? Distance is often measured by driving or bicycling along the route you walked and reading your odometer periodically as you go along. Note the distances by recognizable landmarks so that you can relate them to future walks—note one every half mile or kilometer if possible. Then it is a simple matter to time how fast you walk each kilometer or mile, to keep track of improvements in speed and conditioning.

Nike has developed a remarkable electronic, strap-on monitor with radar-like capabilities that measures speed, distance and your heart rate. It reports information verbally at the touch of a button. Unfortunately, it retails for about $200, but it may well be worth it for some walkers, especially those recovering from heart disease.

Another, but sometimes inaccurate, way to measure distance walked is with a pedometer, a small device you can carry clipped to your belt that is sensitive to the impact of each step you take. It can be adjusted to your stride length. But because of the many variables due to speed and terrain changes, pedometers give only a rough estimate of distance walked and may not be worth the cost.

Just as good is counting the number of paces as measured on a 400-meter track. Walk at your usual exercise rate while counting off quarter-mile segments as you go. Check this periodically as you get into better shape and your speed increases. Orienteers commonly use this technique to find their way and to keep from getting lost around their courses in wilderness or other wooded areas. See the stride-length table on page 186.

Many hiking and biking trails have distances measured along them. If none are available and if there are many exercisers in your area, you might ask the local parks department to provide a measured trail for the citizenry. You'll be surprised what a little lobbying can accomplish. There are estimates that 66 million Americans exercise to some extent at the present time. It is also estimated that a vast majority of them—50 million—are walkers. That should impress local elected officials. If there is a local walking or hiking club, get involved with them and help them lobby for improved facilities. If you are a self-starter, see pages 219–222 for advice on how to start your own club.

Now let's get back to your first walk, your baseline. Dr. Seiden recalls his first measured walk on an indoor track—a mile in 17 minutes. Although he didn't know whether it was good or bad, he felt satisfied with the results. The next day he pushed harder and did a mile in 15 minutes; still feeling OK, he proceeded to do another in 16 minutes. Thirty-one minutes for those two miles gave him a real sense of accomplishment.

We really don't care how fast you go or how far. All that matters is you do it at a comfortable pace. If it takes 20 minutes to negotiate a mile and you feel good at the end, terrific. The speed will increase with time, if you are consistent. Increase either speed or distance as you get in better and better shape. Either way you're improving, and it is faster improvement than you realize.

## The Most Important Thing in Your Life Is Taking Time for Your Health

Now you must begin to schedule your walks. They must be daily! This is vital to your success. If you fail to keep up your walking, you are implying, "Everything I did today is more important than my life and health."

Set a specific time for your walk each day and let nothing impose on that special, top-priority period. We're willing to bet that right about now you're saying, "I don't have the time to permanently schedule a walk."

Oh, yes you do. In fact you can't afford to NOT make the time. Your life depends upon it. Doctors, lawyers, Indian chiefs, CEOs of Fortune 500 companies, mayors of big and little cities, governors, nurses, teachers, bandits, housewives, priests, businessmen—people in all walks of life find time to work out for an hour or more a day. If you truly are motivated and wish to turn your physical condition around, you'll find the time; if you don't, you're just cheating yourself.

Let's take a look at your day. If you sleep about eight out of the 24 hours, that leaves about 16 from which you need to take one or two for yourself.

How about first thing in the morning? Too rushed? Just get up a little earlier. Many people start off their days with a brisk walk at the crack of dawn. "My wife and I get up as the sun breaks over the horizon," a Kansas City physician states. "We walk for an hour to an hour and a half and get our systems in shape for the day. It gives us a chance to talk about anything we want, to plan our days, to solve family, household and office problems. It has opened up a whole new avenue of communication for us. That early, we don't need to worry about the heat of the day while we walk. In the winter it can be cold, but we just bundle up. If the weather is really bad we use our indoor stationary bikes or go to our club and work out. It always amazes us how many other people work out early in the day. We see them at the club and we see them on the street. For us it is the best time."

Not for you? OK. What about mid-morning? This can be an ideal time for housewives, self-employed people, writers, unemployed or retired people, and any others who have a flexible schedule. It's the time of day when facilities and walking trails are least crowded. In the summer it is usually still cool, and in the winter the sun has burned off the chill. The kids are off to school or about their business. If mid-morning fits into your schedule, you are among the lucky ones!

Still not for you? How about a nooner? Lots of people find nooners very refreshing. If you can take a little extra time to exercise during the lunch period, it can be especially beneficial because you are not likely to eat too much. It is now common to see many office people walking leisurely or briskly at this time of day. It works perfectly if you take your lunch, since brown-bagging and walking are natural companions. Simply walk to a comfortable spot to eat, making a picnic of it, and then walk back. Even with a brief rest while you eat you can get in a good 45-minute walk. Get some of your working companions involved. If you can get the boss to go along maybe you can get a little extra time! More and more companies are recognizing the value of exercise for their employees and are building exercise facilities complete with showers. If you are lucky enough to have this advantage, make noon your time for a workout. If you don't have a place to freshen up after your walk and your job requires you to be a fashion plate in the afternoon, just go a little slower so you don't get too bedraggled and sweaty. Slower paces still burn off nearly the same number of calories for the same distance. Then do a cardiovascular workout at a faster pace after work.

Still holding out? How about mid-afternoon? It is a hotter time of day in the summer, but most often the most pleasant time of day in cooler weather. Check to see if it is possible for you to arrive at work earlier to take advantage of this time. Or possibly you can work through lunch, walk in the afternoon and return to work a little later in the day.

Still not right for you? Maybe after work and before dinner would be ideal. You can unwind from the worries and problems of the day, and a workout at this time will dull your appetite. Exercise puts lactic acid into your blood, which works as a natural appetite depressant. The evening meal should be the smallest of the day.

If you haven't gotten in your workout before dinner, then there are a few hours before bedtime. Your workouts may need to be less strenuous at this time, because your supper is digesting, and strenuous exercise just before bedtime raises your metabolism and energy level and makes it hard to go to sleep soon after the walk.

If no time in the day can be worked into your schedule, then you have a motivational problem. No one is so important to the running of the world that he cannot find a time to guard and improve his physical health. During his tenure in office, Richard Lamm, former governor of Colorado, was one of the busiest people in the state, with a long, demanding schedule. He did, however, still find time to get out and run or walk every morning so that he could show up at his office before 8 a.m. refreshed and ready for a day that more often than not went far into the evening hours. If anyone had an excuse to say he was too busy to exercise, it was our good governor.

Besides motivation, the thing that can do more to assure your success is a walking partner. It is far less easy to slough off when someone is expecting you to join him. When you are partly responsible for aiding in another person's workout, you are not as likely to shirk your responsibility. If it is your spouse, you are very lucky. Studies have shown that if your spouse isn't at all sympathetic with your program, there is about an 80 percent chance that you won't stick with it. On the other hand, if your spouse is enthusiastic about it, then your chances approach 100 percent of being successful.

Walking is in fact an excellent family sport. Anyone of any age from toddler on can take part. A family hike combined with a picnic will weld relationships between children and parents, grandparents, relatives, in-laws and outlaws. It can be great fun to carry infants on your walks too.

## Only the Simplest Equipment Is Needed

Good walking shoes are by far the most important item we can name. Dr. Seiden got his favorite pair on sale for $16. Quality shoes may cost anywhere from $30 to $60 or more, but price shouldn't be the main criterion. (See the shoe diagram on page 71.) You absolutely must find a pair that feels great on your feet. If your feet hurt you will not want to walk. Most running shoes have the wrong heels and cushioning for walking. There are, however, some good running shoes that are better for walkers than others. Shop around. Discount stores often carry the more expensive name brands at reduced prices. Look for the following qualities:

1. A shoe that gives good heel stability when the foot lands on the ground. Some running shoes are too "mushy" and allow the foot to roll excessively when the heel lands. This is called pronation, and it causes an unnatural twisting of the leg and puts strain on the knee and hip. Thick soles are not necessary for walking, since one foot or the other is carrying the body weight at all times.
2. The best walking shoes are beveled or rounded up at the back of the heel to help the heel-strike action, and the sole is designed to promote a rocking action as your foot rolls forward to toe push-off.
3. As running shoes get more "high-tech" for running, they are becoming less suitable for serious walking. For example, many of these have the wrong heels and wrong cushioning. Beware of heel counters that curve inward at the top—common in running shoes—since this is counterproductive to the walking motion and can be very irritating to the Achilles' tendon.
4. Make sure that the mid sole is flexible, since the shoe must bend a good deal when pushing off with the toes at the rear of the stride.
5. Make sure that there is ample room in the toe box. There should be about a half inch of space in front of your longest toe. Cramped toes can lead not only to discomfort but also to damaged toenails, blisters and foot strain.
6. Your shoe should be lightweight, with some means of ventilation. Many of the good walking shoes now on the market are all leather, with small ventilation holes on the top.
7. Make sure that the arch support in the shoe is compatible with your foot. It will make a difference whether you have a high or low arch, or flat feet.
8. Walking shoes should not have a knobby tread on the bottoms, but a shallow tread that is slip-resistant and made of hard, wear-resistant rubber. Heavy treads can pick up mud in wet weather.

9. You should feel that your foot is being held and supported firmly but with no uncomfortable pressure points. The shoe should feel snug without pinching, but remember, you don't need nearly the amount of padding in your shoe that a runner needs.

10. Read articles on the latest walking shoes in magazines such as *Walking*. Then go try some of these on at your local athletic shoe outlet. Wear the same type of socks that you will wear when walking.

11. Once you have found your ideal shoe, stick with it. The old saw, "If it ain't broke, don't fix it," is very true in this case. Having more than one brand or style of shoe can be helpful if, for some reason, you develop a sore spot. You can always switch to the other pair.

12. The life of shoes can be extended by using patching compounds designed for this purpose. When the bottom of the shoe wears unevenly—normally at the outside of the heel—it is wise to even things up with Shoe Goo, Sole Patch, Sole Saver or some other material sold for the purpose. Even urethane glue can be a reasonable patching compound. If you don't keep your shoes in repair, you are likely to get some leg strain and ensuing pains from a faulty foot plant. Even a slight out-of-line foot plant can cause problems, but this is easily corrected if you inspect your shoes periodically and repair them when necessary.

Even though many shoe models cost $50 or more, walking is still an inexpensive sport. With proper maintenance, shoes can last a long time if they are quality items in the first place.

Many running shoe companies have now jumped on the bandwagon and are producing shoes specifically for walking. It is impossible for us to recommend a specific brand or model, because such advice would be completely out of date by the time you read this. And everyone's feet are different, anyway. A great deal of research and shoe testing is going on at this point, and many of the new "healthwalkers" seem to be excellent products for their intended purpose. Improved models will continue to show up as time goes by because of the research and development.

Now let's look into the rest of your attire. Compared to shoes, none of the rest of your attire is nearly as important, but we will discuss other items briefly.

1. Socks. These must be snug fitting and free of seams or bumps that might irritate the foot. For normal fitness walking, wear ordinary sweat socks, which can be wool, cotton or a combination of these with nylon. The combinations provide the cushioning plus the absorption of natural fibers and the quick-drying characteristics of the synthetic material.

For long walks there is an advantage to wearing snug, light socks as an inner layer or "second skin," to cut down on friction; for the outer layer, wear socks with a cushioned sole.

2. Shorts should be thin and lightweight material, usually nylon, which is soft and non-chafing to the inner thigh and crotch. Good men's shorts have an inner support of the same material.

3. Cold and foul weather apparel. For cold weather many people are finding that Lycra or polypropylene tights are excellent. And a good windbreaker is essential to keep the chill off. You can get as fancy as you want with Gore-tex and other expensive materials, but this is not necessary unless you want to be a fashion plate.

You lose a great deal of heat through the head, so an ear band or wool hat is a great item to have if it's really cold. The tendency is to overdress rather than underdress, so remember that the body produces a surprising amount of heat in the exercise mode. If you have a cross-country ski outfit, it can be used for winter walks also. Mittens or warm gloves will make the walk far more pleasant, since hands can get cold very quickly unless protected. In extremely cold weather frostbite is a very real consideration, and anyone who has experienced it can attest to the fact that it is very painful.

4. Packs. It is wise to wear a fair-size fanny pack to carry the items that you want to take off if you start to get too warm, or to carry water or snack items, sunglasses, etc. A fanny pack works better than a back pack, which pulls on the upper body and restricts its motions.

5. Time and music. You may wish to use either a digital or sweep-hand wristwatch to keep track of time as you walk.

Watches are very inexpensive these days. Although some people use a "Walkman" for entertainment while they walk, we prefer to enjoy nature on ours. If music motivates you, go ahead and use one but don't let it distract you from the threat of traffic and other dangers.

Realistically speaking, it is the shoes that are of utmost importance. As for the rest, you probably already have enough to "make do" if you wish to get by inexpensively. Anything that is warm and comfortable should suffice.

## Start Healthwalking Now

We have now covered the basic information to help you get going. It is time to take action, but don't do too much too soon. Build up gradually and start working toward personal goals that will enhance your quality of life in future years through healthwalking. Chapter 6 will help you set those goals.

CHAPTER 6

# LITTLE GOALS . . . BIGGER GOALS

*"The more a person is able to direct his life consciously the more he can use time for constructive benefits."*

—Rollo May

---

Your ultimate goal is to increase your life span to its maximum potential and maintain your productivity and activity levels for the duration. You don't want to go out of this life as a fragile, sickly, bedridden and dependent person. Nor do you want to drop dead of a coronary or stroke in the prime of your life and before you reap the harvest of your labors.

Useful longevity is the ultimate goal. To get there you have to set some sub-goals. Your ultimate goal is realistic. Let's make sure the sub-goals are:

1. Over the next few weeks increase your daily walks by at least one mile and shave a minute off your mile time.
2. Find your ideal workout pulse rate and begin to walk at the minimum range level for 45 minutes or longer per day.
3. Set a realistic weight goal for yourself and tune your dietary habits and workouts to attain that goal at more than one pound per week gain or loss, as your case may require.
4. Increase your level to the mid-range pulse level as your strength and endurance increase.
5. Pay attention to and try to break your destructive habits.

6. Increase your performance to the upper ranges of your ideal pulse level.

7. Be in the best shape you've been in in years by the end of the first year of your lifetime walking program.

8. Maintain your health status with the methods we prescribe throughout life, even if it extends for over 100 years.

Go over the following list with your health professional to see if it is realistic for your particular condition. But be as aggressive as possible in your goal setting. You can accomplish more than you think, but only if you work hard at it.

GOAL 1: *Add distance and reduce time from your original baseline level.* Improve from the baseline point established on your first walk, whatever it was. Each day add steps, and as you get stronger, speed those steps up a bit. Improvement will follow improvement. Never slide back! Before you know it, you will be logging miles faster and faster.

When you get to the point where you can walk a mile in about 15 minutes in relative comfort, you'll be ready to move on to the next stage. Then work at lengthening your walks until you can walk four of those 15-minute miles back to back. You will have achieved very good endurance if you can walk four miles in an hour. Then try to walk those miles in 14 minutes each, or the four miles in a brisk 56 minutes.

GOAL 2: *Walk at your minimum ideal pulse rate.* As a general rule, if you can walk even one 14-minute mile without straining, that is what can be defined as a brisk walk. From this point on, unless you want to get into competitive racewalking, we will be less concerned with mile times than with pulse counting. (For those of you interested in racewalking, see Chapter 8.)

Here is how to determine your safe and effective walking pulse rate: The maximum attainable pulse rate for humans is 220. To determine your own safe and effective walking pulse rate, subtract your age (let's say you're 50) from 220:

$$220 - 50 = 170.$$

Therefore 170 is your approximate maximum pulse rate. If .60 represents 60 percent of your maximum heart rate (the generally accepted minimum to achieve a training effect), that means that 170 x .60 is your approximate minimum training rate: 102 pulse beats per minute.

So, if you are 50 years old, you should try to maintain a 45-minute to an hour walk at a speed that will keep your pulse rate at about 100 to 110 beats per minute. After you have been walking for five or 10 minutes, take your pulse at your wrist or the side of the neck. Count the number of beats for six seconds and multiply by 10 (just add a zero to your count). To be slightly more accurate, count the beats for 10 seconds and multiply by six. If your natural pulse rate is unusually fast or slow, you may need to get the guidance of a trained exercise expert to determine your best training range.

Check the calculations of your ideal pulse rates against the table of IPRs on page 184.

If the walking speed that brings you to your minimum ideal pulse rate feels too slow for a comfortable walk, you may need to pick up the pace and walk at the median level as described in Goal 4.

*About warm-ups and cool-downs.* Although we are not enthusiastic about intense warm-ups and a lot of stretching of cold muscles, we do emphatically recommend an adequate cool-down period after a brisk walking session. The cool-down period is very helpful in preventing muscle cramps, stiffness or aches and pains after a workout. There have been cases of cardiac arrest after intense workouts that are abruptly ended without a good cool-down period. Intensive exercise causes enzymes to be released into the bloodstream that can bring on cardiac arrythmias (irregular heartbeats) or tachycardia (excessively rapid heart rate) if circulated while at complete rest. In rare occasions these enzymes can cause fatal cardiac arrest. A cool-down will avoid this problem by burning the enzymes off through gradually diminishing exercise. Joggers and runners are in more danger from this phenomenon than walkers, because their exercise is more strenuous.

A very good cool-down is to gradually reduce your walking speed for the last five minutes of your workout and, while you are still walking, let your pulse rate slow to under 90 beats per minute—a safe range for practically everyone. Then if you wish to do some stretching exercises on your warmed-up muscles, they will be an ideal finish for your daily program. Follow with a nice shower and you'll feel just great for the rest of your day.

GOAL 3: *Determine your ideal weight and diet.* Before you get into your next exercise stage, we will tell you how to establish your ideal body fat percentage (see pages180–194) and the diet necessary to reach and maintain it (Chapter 9). This is probably a new concept to you, and perhaps even to your doctor or health adviser. It eliminates trying to reach an average figure off a weight chart that may be totally unrealistic. There are cases of heavy and muscular pro football players and weight lifters who actually are very low in body fat percentage but who would be classified as grossly obese by standard height-weight tables.

Your ideal body weight takes into account your frame type, muscular build and fat content. It is a dynamic, changing number and may be more or less than you weigh now. Once determined, you will be shown how to reach and maintain it with minimum dietary change—providing your diet is not loaded with all the wrong things.

Within reason, your diet will be built around the foods you like and ones that like you, and deprivation will be avoided as much as practicable. Your diet must be balanced with your activity level and be one you can live with happily for the rest of your life. If arranged correctly, you will never "diet" again but eat sensibly instead.

GOAL 4: *Walk at your mid-range pulse rate.* When you are comfortably able to walk for an hour at your minimum ideal pulse rate, you are ready to advance to working at a higher level. The formula is the same—you just work at a higher percentage of your maximum ideal pulse rate:

$$.70 \times 170 = 119 \text{ (your mid-range IPR)}.$$

As you get in better shape you can exercise safely closer to your maximum heart rate. You should now increase your walking speed to maintain your pulse rate close to 120 beats per minute. When you can do this comfortably for 45 minutes to an hour you will advance to your next stage.

GOAL 5: *Break your destructive bad habits.* Besides getting regular exercise and following a healthy diet, the people who live to the maximum of their life potential actively and productively don't poison their systems with harmful chemicals. So if you smoke, drink too much or indulge in legal or illegal drugs, you absolutely must cut it out. Chapter 10,

"Fight Killer Habits," deals specifically with this problem. Read it if "the shoe fits."

GOAL 6: *Walk at your upper ideal pulse rate.* Using the same formula as before: 220 - 50 = 170 x .80 = 136 (your maximum IPR). From this point on build up your endurance until you can walk 45 minutes to an hour with a steady pulse rate of around 136 beats per minute. This will be your maximum ideal pulse rate from now on if you are 50 years old. This does not mean that you can't improve any more. You will improve considerably from this point. As you get into better and better shape, it will take faster speeds to keep your pulse rate at this level. As your cardiovascular system improves its efficiency, your pulse will begin to slow while doing any given pace so you will have to speed up and expend more energy to keep it at this level. As time goes on, you will not only walk faster but, in going farther in the 45-minute walks, you will be burning off more calories and strengthening your heart, circulatory system and lungs at the same time.

The 170 pulse rate in our 50-year-old example is the maximum attainable heart rate for that age, and is a fairly good approximation for someone of that age. If you exert yourself to the maximum for a short burst, you might approach this level, but you should not do this until you are in very good shape. There is really no good reason to exceed your upper-range IPR unless you are training for serious competition and are doing interval training. As your age increases, each of the IPR levels goes down. Try to stay within your range based on your present age as time goes by. Check your levels against the tables on page 184.

GOAL 7: *A year from now be in the best shape ever.* Unless you have been in very good shape all your life, you can with proper training accomplish this goal. You can have a cardiovascular status and muscle tone better than any you've known in the past. You will be nearer your ideal body weight and have endurance and energy you have never known before. All it takes is dedication and getting out to walk and then walk some more. You will always be glad that you did.

GOAL 8: *Maintain your healthy condition for life.* It is of little benefit to achieve this finely tuned mind and body if it is only temporary. Indeed, it might be harmful to go up and down between good and bad shape. Getting into excellent shape takes a good deal of effort that should not be wasted. Unfortunately, that fitness cannot be stored; it needs to be maintained and nurtured.

Keep in mind the following pointers in your goal-setting project:

1. Set goals that are measurable so that you can monitor your progress. Avoid vague goals such as "getting in shape," since they can't be measured and usually don't motivate. Set realistic goals for such things as weight loss, walking speed and distance, quitting smoking, reducing alcohol intake, etc.
2. Set up small achievable gradual steps toward larger goals. This will make the long-term goals seem more reachable and help avoid discouragement.
3. Set one high goal and one more modest goal that you are absolutely sure you can reach. If you try for immediate perfection you will surely get discouraged. When you surpass your modest goal and strive toward the harder goal, you can feel a sense of accomplishment.
4. Begin on a low-key basis if you are starting from scratch. Remember that it took long years to get out of shape and that you cannot get into really good condition overnight. Patience and persistence are the keys to improvement. Intense workouts in the early stages can be discouraging and can cause injuries, disappointment and great danger of dropping out entirely.
5. Make sure that your family, friends and associates are well aware of your commitment to self-improvement. Then you will be embarrassed if you don't follow through, especially if you have received the moral support of those close to you.
6. Set short-term goals, such as losing a certain number of pounds before your next birthday or a holiday, and use this as a motivational tool to keep going. Do beware of resting on your laurels after short-term goals are reached. Immediately set another short-term goal.
7. If you fail in reaching a goal, don't give up. Consider it a temporary setback and avoid the things that you can identify as causing you to miss your goal.

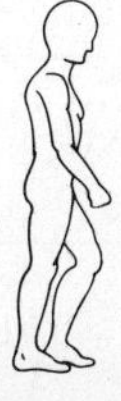

8. If you jot your short- and long-range goals down, they will stay more firmly in mind. Keep track of your successes, of goals met, and this will motivate you to strive for other higher goals to be reached.

Once you have embarked on this program, consider it a lifetime project. It's a new lifestyle for you. Your exercise walking program becomes a daily activity just like eating, sleeping, breathing. Once eliminated, your bad habits should never become a part of your life again. Your new dietary pattern should be no more difficult to maintain than your old one was. If you make it to your goal to be in the best condition you've ever known, you have done the hard part.

CHAPTER 7

# MEASURING YOUR IMPROVEMENT

*"A mile is an exact measure, 5,280 feet. At an average man's walking stride of two feet per step, it will take him 2,640 steps to go the distance. And if he slogs through it counting his steps, it will be a very long mile indeed. But if he goes along interested in what he is seeing, thinking, or talking with a companion, a mile will be hardly any distance at all."*

—Aaron Sussman and Ruth Goode,
Authors of *The Magic of Walking*

---

Whenever we undertake a conditioning program or diet, we tend to step on our scales every day to see what progress we're making. We want you to change this concept. Absolute weight is not the best measure of your progress because so many factors can prompt a temporary change up or down—for example, whether you are very hydrated or dehydrated. If you want to watch your weight fluctuate up or down, OK, but it is not a very important measure of your progress. And do not try to set a designated spot on a standard insurance weight chart as one of your goals. We should try to approach our own ideal body weight, not some average established by insurance company statisticians. After all, the whole purpose of this book is to keep you from becoming a "statistic."

## Your Ideal Body Weight

What is this thing we call "ideal body weight"? That weight that leaves you with the lowest percentage of body fat—it is different for each of us. Let's take an obvious example. Think of a running back on your favorite pro football team. He may

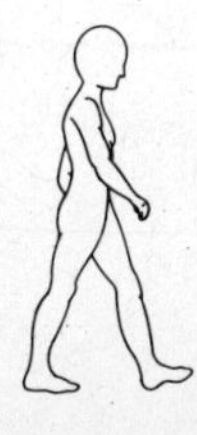

not be a particularly tall man, maybe as short as 5' 9". On a weight chart he would, even under the "large frame" column, be listed as 165 pounds maximum for ideal weight. But, his actual weight may be 210 pounds. He is certainly a finely tuned athlete with a body that is muscular and lean. He actually has a very low percentage of body fat. He has very nearly approached his ideal body weight. But the weight chart says that he is drastically overweight. He certainly could not do his job on the football team if he weighed that "ideal weight." Yet he might have difficulty buying life insurance because of "obesity." After all, the weight chart says to the insurance company that he probably, because of excess weight, is likely to have more than normal health problems.

Let's carry this example further to see how fallacious the weight charts can be. Let's assume our running back wants that insurance policy so badly he is willing to comply and reach his designated level on the weight chart. He decides to lose the requisite 45 pounds. To do it he must lose all his excess fat, of which there is very little—maybe less than 8 or 10 percent. The bulk of the 45 pounds will need to come from eliminating healthy muscle and glandular tissue. This would not only be extremely difficult but also unhealthy and patently absurd.

We can conclude, then, that weight charts are not the measure that we should use. The concept of ideal body weight, an individualized figure for each of us, is far more sensible.

Your ideal body weight can fluctuate—it is not a constant. You may have had a relatively high percentage of body fat when you started your walking program, especially if you were somewhat sedentary. As you walk faster and farther, you will not only burn off some of that excess fat but you will also tone and put on some healthy muscle tissue. Adding and toning muscle tissue in itself reduces the percentage of fat weight that makes up your total body weight. So as you work out, and your weight goes down somewhat, your ideal body weight figure and actual weight approach each other. As you get in better shape, you might find that you don't need to lose all the weight you originally set as your goal. Isn't that a pleasant thought?

What if you are underweight? Slimness is admired in the USA, but it can be carried too far. The solution for underweights is not much different than that for overweights. As you work out, you too will tone and add muscle mass. Muscle weighs more than fat, and so your exercise walking program may actually cause you to gain weight. Overeating is not the solution to being underweight—proper eating is! The correct diet, which will give you the raw materials to build the healthy tissue, is no different from that outlined in the next chapter. As you work out, your ideal body weight and your actual body weight will approach each other, but from different directions.

## Body Measurements

Your tailor will be the first to know. As you work out, you will tone your muscles and lose some of that sag. Your total body weight can actually increase due to building of new muscle tissue, but you may appear to be losing weight and you will look better and healthier. You might even be asked if you are losing weight when you are actually gaining a few pounds. Your belt might require new holes punched as inches start to come off your belly. Your chest may enlarge a bit as your lungs and muscles expand. You might need a larger shirt and smaller belt, skirt or slacks.

Take a few baseline measurements to help you watch the progress. Measure around your chest at the nipple line, around your waist at the belt line, around your hips at the widest point and around your thighs and calves at their largest points. Remeasure each month and keep track of the results. You'll be pleasantly surprised, because the fat and pudge will come off, and hard muscle will replace it as ideal and total body weight approach each other. Then watch your progress as you enter the changing figures over time. This can be very motivating if you keep on the program consistently enough to improve on a gradual basis.

## Resting Pulse Rate

Resting pulses are a measure of your cardiac efficiency and are perhaps your most important indicator. The best time to take your resting pulse is when you are awakening in the morning, before you do anything. It is also possible to take it during the day after sitting completely relaxed for about 10 or

15 minutes, but it will be slightly higher than first thing in the morning. Seiden's pulse before getting into exercise walking was 70 beats per minute, which is considered average. In a few weeks it dropped to about 62 and then gradually to 54, where it is at a steady basis now. That amounts to about a 30 percent drop. This created a large gain in cardiac efficiency. Carlson had a similar experience, except his went from 60 to 42.

Some believe that we have an allotted number of heartbeats in a normal lifetime. It's probably not as simple as that, but if even only partially true, a heart that beats 50 or 60 times a minute should last a lot longer than one that beats 70 to 80 or higher. The longer your ticker runs, the longer you'll be around. Dr. Seiden personally checked the pulses of more than 200 Indians remarkable for their rugged longevity in the Andes Mountains. As a rule, their active pulses ranged around 60 to 70 and the resting rate was 50 and lower. If you wish to purchase a pulse monitor, the Accusplit 161 is the best we have seen for the price.

## Blood Pressure

This is very important to your health and longevity. In the 200 Indians checked in the Andes of Ecuador, there were NO cases of hypertension. Exercise walking, proper diet and elimination of toxic chemicals such as smoking, excess alcohol and drugs are by far the most effective of antihypertensives. The proper walking program alone can bring your blood pressure down by twenty points at both the high and low readings. This is true partially because walking is such a great stress reducer, and it also helps to dilate your vascular system and make it more elastic and responsive to your body's needs. Proper diet and elimination of chemical abuse will help over and above the effects of walking.

## Increased Endurance

If you are consistent, it won't be long until you find yourself breezing through times and distances you found challenging just weeks before. Whether you measure the time it takes you to walk a mile, how many miles you can walk or your ideal pulse rate, you will find rapid improvements in the beginning. The lower the base you start from, the more the improvements will be. These are indications of a generally better-functioning body.

## Feeling Better, Greater Self-Confidence

Shortly after you get into your walking program, you will find that you are feeling better generally. You will have fewer aches and pains, headaches and back problems. You will have more energy, less insomnia, fewer colds and illnesses. Your mood and self-esteem will improve, and depressions will tend to melt away. You will have changed a downhill slide into a new beginning. You will think you're a new and different person—and you really will be. You will have a new lease on life, enjoying pleasure from that life and a longer, brighter future ahead.

You will find that you begin to look better, feel better and think better and more positively. You'll also think better of yourself, as will others. With that will come a renewed boost in your self-confidence. This turnaround in your conditioning and well-being cannot help but cause a tremendous change in the attitude of a person who has been running down and then suddenly begins on an exhilarating uphill course.

## A Greater Degree of Happiness

You cannot help but be happier when you feel better, gain self-respect, and have more energy and endurance. Particularly when others are telling you how much better you look! You will start enjoying life more. Most of your worries and stresses will begin to melt away. Walking does that for you. As all these other things start working for you, you will be pleasantly surprised as your priorities begin to change. Life will be more fun for you, and little things that have been bothering you will become unimportant in your new scheme of things.

These are the important criteria for measuring your progress. If you want to step on a scale once in a while, go ahead. As you keep walking, measure your improvement—there will be a great deal of self-satisfaction as you get better and better in the multitude of ways you have read about in this book.

CHAPTER 8

# RACEWALKING

*"Racewalkers are part of a groundswell that may become the wave of the future. The racewalker, for one thing, can make do with very ordinary feet. He can put miles and miles on feet that would break down in any other sport. And he isn't likely to get injuries farther up in the kinetic chain that goes from foot to leg to knee to thigh to low back. Racewalking is virtually injury free."*

—George Sheehan, M.D.,
Author of *Dr. Sheehan on Running*

---

For the uninitiated among you who may be intimidated by the term "racewalking," let us assure you that it is only a speeded up version of healthwalking. We have discovered that people of all ages can easily pick up the basics of the technique in a very short time. The technique has been developed over the years to make rapid walking as fast and efficient as possible with a minimum of wasted movements. We think that young and old alike among you should become acquainted with the basics to see how you like the feeling of walking fast efficiently.The racewalkers in our Front Range Walkers club range in age from seven to 78 years of age.

In racewalking, older people can compete with younger people for a far longer period than they can in distance running—the gap does not widen nearly as fast. It is not uncommon for people to continue to set personal records at 50 or 60 or even older as they gain in technical efficiency and experience. In distance running, high aerobic capacity is much more of a factor. It is a great ego builder for the aging, walking athlete to be competitive right into his or her later years. In his mid-40s, Larry Walker of Southern California is among the country's elite racewalkers.

One of the things that makes racewalking fun is that the technique is something you can work on and improve each time you go out for a walk, as long as you know what you are working toward. If you walk with a partner, you can help each other detect inefficiencies and faults. We are thoroughly convinced that it is about the best way to get a total-body aerobic workout—better and safer than jogging, organized aerobics or practically any other exercise you can name. At first you may feel that racewalking movements are exaggerated and ungainly, but don't be self-conscious, because the technique looks very powerful and efficient when done correctly, with no side sway or up and down movements. Besides, more and more of your peers are out there doing it and having a ball.

All indicators are now showing that the sport is growing like wildfire nationwide. Notice how all the running shoe companies are jumping on the bandwagon with a plethora of new walking shoes showing up in the marketplace. Also notice the attention walking is getting in all the media, and how many running races now are including walking in their event. Why not heed Dr. Sheehan's advice and join the wave of the future?

Not more than two decades ago, anyone who was over 60, 50 or even 40 years of age was considered to be eccentric, peculiar or downright weird if they trained and competed in endurance sports such as running or racewalking. After all, those sports were supposed to be strictly the domain of the young and vigorous. Obviously (or so they thought in those days), anyone over 40 surely would be inviting a fatal heart attack if they participated in anything more strenuous than bowling or golf. What a difference a few short years make! Now there is a Senior Olympics that is limited to those 55 and over and in which older athletes compete against each other in five-year age groups. Just because you were born a long time ago does not mean that an urge to compete does not still swell in your breast. There are those who pursue physical excellence no matter how old they are getting chronologically.

Age-group awards for those over 40 in racing make competitors anticipate getting into the next-older age classification—which can have quite a profound effect on the ability to win. This can remove a lot of the stigma of getting older, and most certainly add to enthusiasm to participate. It gives an incentive to work toward getting in better and better physical condition as the five- or ten-year milestones (not millstones) of age classification are passed—milestones that we used to hate to admit to anyone. Entering the next decade is not so painful at all in the minds of aging competitors, since they then become the "new kids on the block."

Following is a tale most will find hard to believe, as was true in our case until we actually met him. It is about Gordon Wallace of Prescott, Arizona. In 1976, Gordon, at age 66, was faced with severe coronary artery disease, and he underwent a triple-bypass operation to alleviate the condition. Subsequently, he had the choice of following the usual medical management—featuring drugs and a sedentary lifestyle—or of undertaking a moderate regimen of progressive exercise. He chose the latter and he faced the challenge with confidence.

He changed his diet to a near-vegetarian type, as he had been convinced that high cholesterol had been the main culprit in causing his illness. After three months of carefully monitored exercise and diet, he was taking extended hikes in the mountains. He then began experimenting with all sorts of aerobic exercises—swimming and then jogging (both of which he thought too tedious) and finally racewalking, which he found to be the perfect exercise for him. He has had no symptoms of his former disease since starting his walking program. Within four years, after training diligently, he was competing in and winning world championships in his age division. He is holder of 25 American age-group records; was named national masters racewalker of the year in 1980 and 1981, world champion at 5 kilometers and 20 kilometers in 1981, champion at European Veterans Championships in 1980, and outstanding masters athlete at Pan American Masters Games in 1981; and has received other honors too numerous to mention here. As you will note, some of his most fantastic achievements came only four years after his coronary bypass operation. He continues to compete vigorously on a world-class level to this day.

Gordon is obviously not your typical heart patient because of his extreme dedication to physical fitness, but if others would follow his path as described in his book, *The Valiant Heart:From Cardiac Cripple to World Champion*, even on a modest scale, there would be far fewer cardiac and other medical problems in our country today. He says: "The basic elements of my attitude include the welcome of a challenge, a 'can-do' mentality, adherence to the maxim, 'God helps those who help themselves,' and the absence of fear in living my life." He is truly an inspiration to anyone of any age—and all his successes came from his regimen of rapid walking in the racewalking style.

## Some Walking History

In this country we are now experiencing an unprecedented rise in the popularity of racewalking. Actually, racewalking was very popular in this country and in England in the latter part of the 19th century, when it was called "pedestrianism." The races ranged from an hour or two- to six-day events and even walks for thousands of miles across the country. (The most famous racewalker of the time was our American champion Edward Payson Weston, whose career started just prior to the Civil War and lasted until the late 1920s, when he was struck down by a taxi at age 88, at which time he was still walking remarkable distances. He died two years later from the injuries sustained in this unfortunate accident.)

The best walkers turned professional, and large sums of money were wagered on the outcome of events. The contestants were amply compensated as well. Some marks were set that seem excellent to this day. What makes some of the records even more amazing is the fact that the participants wore ordinary (or even stylish) clothing and did not have the high-tech, lightweight shoes that aid today's athletes. However, the sport sank almost out of sight in the early 20th century and remained there until about 1970, when it started to re-emerge. The Olympic Games did include the sport during those "dark ages" from 1908 on, thus keeping the sport alive but, nevertheless, fairly obscure.

Today, our favorite Colorado racewalker is Viisha Sedlak. At age 39 she is one of the best woman ultramarathoners in the world and a U.S. National team member in racewalking. At the world championships in La Rochelle, France, in October 1985, she completed her first six-day race and finished fourth. In this race she used the technique of interspersing fast walking with running, and thereby spread the load of the exercise over more muscles of the body than just the legs. The running muscles received some rest during the walking periods. Required medical tests were performed on each contestant at the end of the race. Viisha was informed that she was the least injured of all the athletes in the race, due to the fact she had combined the two disciplines much more than the others. In December 1987 she won two gold medals in racewalking at the World Veterans' Championships in Australia.

Both of us (the authors) and Rob Sweetgall, who walked 11,208 miles through all 50 states in 50 weeks in 1985, can attest to the fact that long distances are best covered by walking than running, especially if you want to avoid trauma.

## Is Racewalking for Me?

Do you wonder if or why racewalking is going to be good for you personally? Let's take a look at some of the specifics of the sport. The technique of racewalking allows exercisers to get the maximum ambulatory speed possible short of running. There are two rules that differentiate racewalking from running. One is that one foot or the other must be in contact with the ground at all times. That is, the front heel must strike the ground before the rear toes leave it. If both feet are off the ground at any one time, the competitor is violating the "lifting" rule. Lifting does not ordinarily occur except at the walker's maximum speed or unless he or she is jogging.

The other rule is that the competitor must straighten his leg to a straight or locked-knee position at mid-stride as the leg passes beneath the trunk. Watch an old Marx Brothers movie sometime and you will see Groucho giving a comical demonstration of the violation of this rule. Leg straightening is really the only basic difference between racewalking and ordinary strolling, although, if you watch closely, many people naturally straighten their legs even during slow walks. The leg muscles must pull the body forward, starting from a position at heel strike slightly in front of the body and progressing to a straight leg at the rear. This gives the feeling of pulling the ground surface beneath you as you move along. If the legs do not straighten, the violation is called "bent knee." Maximum efficiency is gained if the leg is straight throughout the stride from heel strike to toe lift-off.

Racewalking can be a very technical sport for those who seek excellence and proficiency. Casual walkers need not worry a great deal about the finer points in technique, but many of the suggestions here can help make walking more enjoyable and efficient.

## A Challenge for Life!

In a few weeks almost anyone who gets a little instruction can learn reasonable and efficient form. It can take years, though, to develop a flawless form such as some of the champions have. This fact may be more of an advantage than a disadvantage, since it gives a person a challenge every time out to think about and improve efficiency little by little during each practice session. For those of you who do have a competitive bent, the physical benefits of speedwalking or racewalking are like those of long-distance running.

Good racewalkers have startling endurance. Walking at speed strengthens all the leg muscles—the flexor muscles of the hip, the stomach muscles and the muscles in the lower back. In addition, rapid walking produces a considerable mobility in the shoulders, trunk, hips and ankles. All of these actions are important to older people, since lack of use and mobility are what cause them to become decrepit before their time. Runners must, on the other hand, commonly do supplementary exercises to develop muscles of the upper body.

We would like to interject the idea that racewalking should be synonymous with health and fitness walking, because the correct form utilizes and strengthens more of the body's total muscular system than practically any other exercise that you could name. Therefore even if you aren't interested in racing, the racewalking form is the best muscle toner of any sport outside of cross country skiing. Actually the two are closely related because both are gliding movements, and both use a greater number of muscles than nearly any other exercise. RACEWALKING IS JUST AS AEROBICALLY BENEFICIAL AS RUNNING AND JOGGING.

Howard Jacobson, renowned coach in New York City and

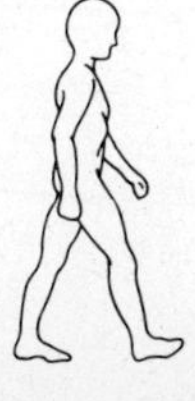

author of *Racewalk to Fitness*, suggests that a good workout is to walk 11 to 13 minutes per mile, depending on personal condition, for about 30 minutes per session. He finds race-walking a good exercise for firming and strengthening the buttocks and thighs, because the heel hits the ground first, activating the buttock and then the thigh muscles to pull the body over the leg. The muscles of both the front and back of the legs are consciously and deliberately used, thus creating a balanced muscle tone not applicable to running.

## Practice and Patience Make Perfect

Let's discuss some of the elements that lead toward an efficient style. If you wish to learn to walk fast efficiently, it is essential that you learn and practice form correctly from the beginning. Do not attempt to walk too fast initially—the ability to walk with the best efficiency will not happen immediately. At first, you may feel that the correct form is slower than natural rapid hiking pace, but as technique improves, so will speed and efficiency. Until form becomes somewhat automatic, it is necessary to concentrate. Be aware of a posture that will constantly maintain or improve forward progression and proper body balance whether you are walking uphill, downhill or on the level. Maintain an upright body position with your hips directly under the upper body. Try to get the feeling of sitting on the hips. A slight lean of about 5 percent forward from the ankles is good for purposes of maintaining momentum, but leaning too far forward will shorten the stride and put strain on the hamstring muscle. Stand up straight with no bending at the waist, and keep the head up at all times—don't let the chin drop toward the chest, since this will reduce breathing capacity and cause tenseness and fatigue.

Flexibility and relaxation of the hips is all-important since it allows the necessary rolling, dropping and twisting movements for moving the legs quickly and efficiently. Avoid overstriding, using a bent-legged, non-hip rotating hiking style. Good stride length will be achieved with the correct hip-rolling, leg-straightening style, which in the long run is the only way to maintain efficient and rapid leg movement. Rotate the hips from front to back with very little side movement.

Place the leading foot down directly in front of the trailing one so that they are in a straight line. Increased flexibility in the hips and mid-section will increase stride length. Strong twisting action of the stomach, hips, lower back and waist allows you to go faster with less effort and strain on the legs. Swing the front leg in front, landing on the heel, and pull the knee back in a straightened, locked position. If you overstride and put the heel too far in front, there will be a braking action until you pull yourself over the pulling leg. Try to rotate your hip as far as possible over the leading leg during heel strike. Concentrate on keeping the leg straight as you pull it back. Pulling with a straight leg aids in the hip rotating and twisting action, and adds speed and smoothness to forward progress.

Follow through with the pulling action of the straight leg by rolling off the foot on the toes. As the body weight is pulled forward, it rolls across the outside edge of the foot to all the toes. The foot acts like a rocking chair so that no one part of the structure takes the entire weight of the body for more than an instant. When the trailing leg leaves the ground and swings forward, the knee bends just enough to allow the foot to skim barely above the ground as it passes beneath the body. As the heel lands, the toes should be pointed upward and straight ahead; splaying the toes out is very inefficient. Avoid rolling on the inside of the foot, since this may cause pain and eventual injury. For best efficiency, the feet should just skim above the surface of the ground as they are in the swing phase. The swing phase allows the leg to relax before pressure on the ground is applied in the next stride.

There should be a conscious attempt to keep the rear foot on the ground as long as possible to take advantage of a powerful thrust of all the toes as they leave the ground. The fastest walkers in the world are now concentrating on this thrust from as far back as possible to get maximum power from their stride. This factor, along with hyperextension of the rear leg, is what gives them their startling efficiency and speed. This takes extreme hip flexibility and is only gained through years of practice. In walking, the pulling/pushing foot is on the ground for over two-thirds of the time, while in running it is on the ground one-third of the time or less, depending on speed and stride length.

The arms are moved as in normal walking, close to the body. swinging counter to the legs, and are bent at a 90-degree angle. Let the hands move naturally to the middle of the chest but no higher than the breastbone, since higher may lift you off the ground. Vigorous arm and shoulder motion exercises the muscles of the arms, shoulders, chest and back. Pull the elbow back but then relax the muscles and let gravity pull the hands to a position four inches in front of the breastbone. Ideally the arms should move in an elliptical motion—hands "scooping" low past the hips then curling up toward the chest. This motion causes a shoulder prop, which indirectly aids in stride efficiency and speed. Keep the elbows as close as possible to the body as they swing past. Do not hunch the shoulders up, because that will tighten the neck and shoulder muscles, waste energy and cause tiredness sooner. When walking slowly to warm up or cool down, the arms may be held lower, with the elbows at a more open angle, but always swinging briskly to get the full benefit of the exercise. Holding the arms too far down at the side will cause blood to pool in the fingers, producing swelling; and in that position the pendulum of the arm motion is too long and, therefore, slow.

We must now interject absolutely the most important point of all: The more relaxed you are as you do any of the described movements—whether in the legs, upper body or arms—the faster you will progress and the more efficient you will become. In addition, all of the foregoing words of advice are not as complicated as they sound since they are the prerequisites for higher speeds and will happen automatically as speed is increased to about 5 mph or faster, as long as you have a basic idea of correct technique and apply it.

## Little by Little Your Style Will Develop

Have fun working on the components of good style by working on one thing at a time until perfected, then move to the next. You will feel it when things fall into place and efficiency and speed improve. The techniques of good posture, hip rotating, pulling back straight-legged, proper foot roll and arm pumping are the same for everyone. As you gain flexibility and strength in the motions and positions of this healthful

1. Hips drop and roll while twisting back and forth. This allows your legs to move faster and easier and gives you a longer stride. Note how stripe on side of shorts moves from front to rear.
2. Arms always bent at a 90-degree angle and pumped vigorously. Let hands swing to the center of your chest as they move back and forth.
3. Knee bends as leg is swung forward. This allows toes to clear ground.
4. Knee straightened all the way back at this point and pulling ground as heel touches.
5. Toes and calf muscles push body forward. Feet land on a straight line with toes pointed directly forward.
6. Keep neck and shoulders relaxed.
7. Body and head in upright position at all times. Always concentrate on correct technique. This helps time and effort pass quicker and makes you feel and look better.

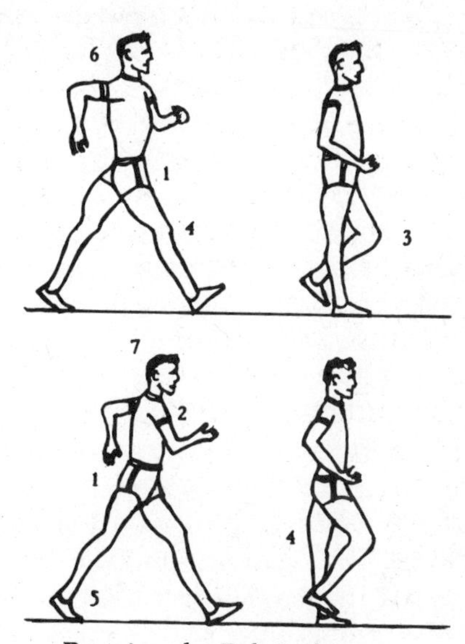


*—Drawings by Bob Carlson*

exercise, you will develop a style that is smooth and naturally suited to your unique body build and current level of fitness. You will begin to feel rhythm and ease as the ground flows below—you will be moving with the same sense of confidence and grace that a champion racewalker experiences.

Walking with hip rolling eliminates the rise and fall of the trunk. You will see hikers, and others who are trying to walk fast without using the hip motion of racewalking, bounding up and down to some extent. This is a waste of energy if you are trying to walk fast efficiently.

You don't have to lift your weight off the ground as you do in running, so it allows people of different builds and weights to compete fairly equally. Distance runners, to be really good, should be in the 120- to 140-pound range if short, and in the 140- to 160-pound range if tall. It is possible for heavier and more muscular exercisers to do better in walking, comparatively speaking, since they can "power their way along" against the resistance that is inherent in keeping one foot on the ground at all times.

## Running vs. Walking

Bob Carlson has competed in a vast number of both running and racewalking events, and has some basic observations on the two sports and how they are viewed by the participants. There are some misconceptions that participants who have not tried both have about each other's sport. Runners seem to think that racewalking is very hard as they see the swinging of the arms, shoulders and hips in the characteristic exaggerated fashion. To a walker the running looks relatively easy if the runner they are watching is using an efficient and economical style. Each perception is equally wrong. Both competitors are putting in about the same amount of effort as their particular conditioning allows. The mode of progression dictates the apparent energy output. The great amount of energy the runner is expending is disguised by the fact that the runner is putting a tremendous amount of effort into the springing action of his legs, and mostly this action only. A racewalker must remain in contact with the ground, and to overcome this factor he quickens and lengthens his stride. The quickness of his movement is counterbalanced by equally rapid arm action and shoulder movements. A world-champion walker can achieve a stride rate of 31/2 steps per second or more when moving at full speed. The quest for a longer stride gives him a very observable hip rolling action not seen in any other sport.

Upper body power is more important to a walker than a runner—a strong motor (heart) in a light frame is vital to a distance runner who wants to do well. A factor in the walker's favor is that he gets tired gradually and can walk a little slower without altering his basic form, style and rhythm. On the other hand, when fatigue strikes a runner, it can strike very rapidly and he can be reduced to a slow shuffle in a very short time. When a running competitor is really washed out or has "hit the wall," it is extremely difficult or even impossible to run with any authority at all, which can be a very pathetic sight. Walkers, no matter how tired, can normally still move along, however slowly, with some semblance of their normal competitive form.

Dr. Tom DeLauro, dean of the New York College of Podiatric Medicine, says that even though some soreness is almost certain to occur during the first couple of weeks of racewalking, injuries serious enough to prevent further training very rarely occur. He does recommend stretching exercises of both the front and back muscles of the leg before and after training to loosen them up. He also recommends straightening the leg with a natural relaxed movement rather than snapping the knee back hard on each step at first, until the knee muscles and tendons become very well conditioned. Most beginners tend to feel soreness in the foot elevator muscles, which makes the shin feel sore—a feeling akin to shin splints. This is because there is an increased range of motion in the stride length, and the toes must be lifted by certain muscles on each stride to keep them from dragging on the ground. These muscles are not heavily used normally, but can be conditioned by racewalking. Some hip and shoulder soreness may also occur initially, but these will soon disappear after a little training using the correct form.

Bob Carlson, who has never had the slightest injury from walking but has suffered several hamstring and calf pulls from running, believes that there is a great difference in the injury potential of the two. Walkers just seem to go on and on training without injury. But a running injury can be traumatic, causing a layoff from training for an extended period of time. It seems that elite runners must accept injuries as a part of their sport. But a walker is far less likely to have an injury bad enough to disrupt training for more than a few days, and this is rare, even at world-class levels. If a walker has excellent form, he does not have to be in quite as good shape as a runner at the same level to be competitive as he gets older. A lot of this has to do with the foot-pounds of energy necessary to lift the body off the ground in running.

Here are some lessons learned from personal experience: After each of 28 running marathons, Bob was tired and stiff for most of the week afterward. Conversely, after 50k and 30k walking competitions, he felt nearly normal in the next day or two. It could be that racewalking distributes the load of the exercise over a far greater number of muscles, and thus does not put quite as much strain on any of them. On one walk of 50 miles in just over 12 hours, Dr. Seiden was able to go out to dinner two hours later and the next day was free of aches, pains or fatigue. Walking is simply the most natural means of moving the human body from one place to another, and amazing feats of endurance are possible.

Running and jogging may seem more natural to the beginner. More concentration is needed in the initial stages of learning the racewalking technique—but the efficient racewalking movements become nearly automatic with practice. Efficient technique, we repeat, is not learned overnight, and persistence is all-important. Although the same aerobic benefits are attained in racewalking as in running, it is far more of a challenge to learn and a whole lot more fun.

## It's Not as Funny-Looking as Some Think

There are plenty of "unnatural"-looking movements connected with many different activities that do not draw much attention. There are track and field events such as the shot put, triple jump, discus, high jump, etc., that are learned skills and are not what you would call "natural movements" but that are unique to those events. No one gives these movements a second thought because they are necessary to achieve good results. Considering this, it is unfortunate that the extremely beneficial and necessary hip swiveling action of racewalking is considered to be strange by vast numbers of the uninformed public. Actually, the correct form looks powerful and efficient. Certainly, fellow track athletes respect the effort required to become a good racewalker, because the necessary dedication is similar to their own.

Those who have never exerted themselves in their life by walking at faster than a casual stroll perhaps don't realize that, in order to gain real walking speed practically all of the muscles of the body must come into play. Of course, the unusual movements are precisely what make racewalking the complete and perfect exercise it is. This sort of misunderstanding by the general public is the biggest drawback to the success of racewalking as a sport in the USA. The sport is much bigger in Europe, where it is more fully understood. Fortunately, the tide is now turning. Walking is now being touted by the various media as the best exercise for the greatest number of people because of its injury-free characteristics and superior total body toning.

## Walking Shoes vs. Racing Shoes

Shoes are indeed important for speedwalkers as they are for any walker. Racewalkers do not need nearly as much padding as joggers and runners because the weight is always on one foot or the other.We include here a diagram of the essentials of a good speedwalking (or healthwalking) shoe.

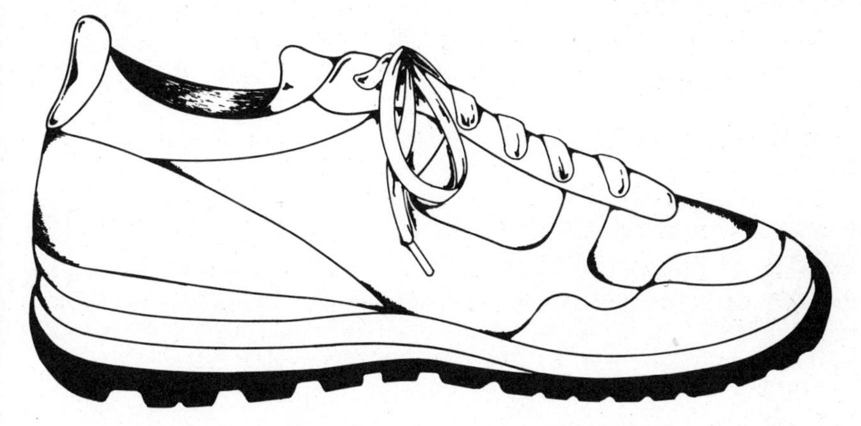

A great boon to the promotion of racewalking is the newly formed North American Racewalking Foundation in Pasadena, California, with John McLachlan as founder and chairman and Elaine Ward as managing director. For many years, Elaine and John have been extremely active in providing information, development and promotion of racewalking. If you wish to know how to get advice or how to get started, refer to the section on "Useful Information for Walkers" for a list of clubs and individuals throughout the country who put on events and instructional clinics in their particular areas. They all welcome newcomers and offer encouragement. We also list a Bibliography of other helpful books on the subjects of racewalking or healthwalking in general. So for those of you who can make the effort to get into very good condition, have a competitive nature and wish to test yourself, racewalking may be just the answer to keep the spring in your legs, a twinkle in your eyes and a smile on your face as you speedwalk through life.

## CHAPTER 9

# YOUR HEALTHY DIET

*"Many programs fail simply because the person doesn't have a strong enough desire to lose weight by eating less or exercising more."*
—Dr. Joyce Brothers

---

Why are the bookstores loaded with diet books of every conceivable type? Ironically, it is probably because most of these diets don't work. People who are looking for easy ways to lose weight tend to try one diet after another, seeking the ideal one—and all the while the book sales are booming. The truth is that the ideal diet is seldom found, and even if it were it would not be enough. Dieting MUST be accompanied by suitable exercise to be truly effective, and to ignore the exercise is a big mistake. It is possible to lose excess weight fast initially through a calorie-restricted diet, but such diets are not pleasant, and cheating usually occurs. After a period of time the excess pounds reappear as if by magic—plus a few extras!

Since there is general agreement among diet authorities that it is counterproductive to lose more than about a pound a week, we do not recommend the crash or fad diets that get a lot of publicity and are advertised heavily. We are violently opposed to fad diets of any kind. Here we will guide you as simply as possible to the correct foods to eat and to the avoidance of foods that have a detrimental effect on the human body.

It seems strange, but it is true that moderate exercise will actually decrease appetite. Combining exercise with a sensible diet will result in the loss of 80 percent fat instead of equal loss of fat and muscle tissue on a low-calorie diet without exercise. Exercise allows you to take in more calories each day, and because of this it is much easier to obtain the minimum daily requirements of more essential vitamins and minerals. In addition, since our bodies were designed to be exercised, it is really very difficult for most people to maintain their ideal body weight without it. Have you noticed the plethora of pot bellies carried around by your sedentary friends and associates? It is like an epidemic, especially in men, and so easily avoided through sensible exercise. Brisk walking is the best way to trim off extra inches of girth and pounds and to keep them off through life.

If you didn't change your diet in any way and just added brisk walking for an hour a day to your routine, you would lose almost a pound a week just from the 2,800 or so additional calories you would be burning off. A pound is worth about 3,500 calories. This means that you could conceivably lose nearly 50 pounds in a year without any diet change at all.

One of the benefits of a vigorous walking program is that it develops strong muscles in the arms and shoulders—strong enough to push you away from the table before you overeat. We often eat more than we need—we eat things because they taste too good to quit. This is common in fast eaters. Try to be a fast walker and a slow eater. Talk at the table and make it a social event, not a competitive event to see who gets seconds first. Drink a lot of water during the meal. Take small bites and savor each one, chewing thoroughly. It is amazing how large a mouthful a fast eater can swallow. If the same amount of food were taken in two mouthfuls and thoroughly chewed, it would give you twice the pleasure and fewer calories in the long run (or walk).

Can walking burn as many calories as running? Surprisingly, the answer is YES. Walking can be as hard as you want to make it. If you truly push yourself, you can burn as many calories, or even more, as in running. Fast walking is a TOTAL body exercise, using the upper body to a marked degree as well as the legs. At high speeds it is less efficient than running, in

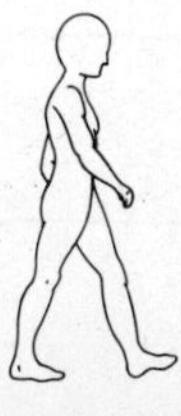

terms of movement, but more efficient in burning calories. The extra effort required in brisk walking adds up to more calories burned for the distance covered.

## Fad Diets

A walking program combined with sensible eating habits—not semi-starvation—is all you need to get your weight to where you want it. To be truly healthy, it is necessary to have a combination of aerobic exercise and healthy nutrition—neither will suffice alone. It is only logical that an ardent exerciser can put away more calories than his sedentary counterpart. It is not how little you eat that will make the difference, but how well you balance the intake and the burning of calories.

We repeat: Beware of fad diets and of other far-out and effortless ways to shed pounds. Regardless of what those who promote body wraps, magic potions and extracts for weight loss say, if you want to lose weight, calories eaten must be fewer than calories burned. Diuretics, steam, perspiration enhancement, wrappings to squeeze water out of your cells are all dehydration methods that are temporary at best and dangerous at worst. As soon as you can get to a water cooler, your cells will reabsorb fluids lost in this manner, and your only permanent weight loss will occur in your wallet.

Furthermore, a diet that reduces your daily caloric intake too much will not let you get the nutritionally balanced diet you need. It is virtually impossible to get a proper diet while following a drastic, calorie-restricted diet, which is what many sedentary people resort to to lose their fat. Many of these fad diets are dangerous to your health. Some have you eating only protein. Some are deficient in dietary fiber. Some are liquids only. Others have you eating concoctions that leave you with a starvation program for weeks on end. None of these restricted diets allows for the nutritionally balanced diet that every living animal needs for good health.

There are no circumstances under which starvation is healthy. It destroys healthy muscular, organ and bone tissue as well as reduces storage fat. Put those fad and starvation diets completely out of your mind and concentrate on the healthy foods that you need for a balanced diet.

There are probably more charlatans preying on the gullible in relation to diet and weight loss than on any other subject. Pick up practically any newspaper or magazine and you will find ads on how to dissolve fat from your body effortlessly while you rest, by eating grapefruit, taking "reducing" pills or wrapping your body like a mummy for an hour or two. Many of these claims are patently ridiculous—yet people still fall for them and spend millions of dollars on them annually. Hopefully we can give sufficient, factual information so you can pick a healthy course of nutrition for yourself—to help you walk away from unhealthy diets and unnecessary dieting.

## Walk Away Those Extra Pounds

What we would like to see happen to you who need to reduce is exemplified by a true story that may give you inspiration. Edmond Rivet, a neighbor of Bob Carlson's, and a teacher in the Cherry Creek school district in suburban Denver, was a rotund fellow in his mid-thirties, stretching to all of 5' 6" and weighing 240 pounds. He had been inactive and a heavy eater. He had tried all the fad diets to no permanent avail. He would go up and down in weight (mostly up), but never seemed to find an effective way to achieve permanent weight loss. He was about to give up, convinced that he was just meant to be fat.

One day while lamenting that it was his lot in life to be overweight, Bob coaxed him into trying a walking program to lose weight. "You mean, all I have to do is walk? I don't have to run and work out daily in a gym? And I don't need to starve myself? I don't see how it could work for me."

Bob finally got him to try to give it a month's honest effort. He started getting out before breakfast each morning. He became consistent and persistent. Although he could not cover much ground at first, after a couple of weeks he was able to cover two miles without undue effort. He became more enthusiastic about this "magic" walking program. He then speeded up a little at a time and got much faster in the course of a few weeks. Then he increased the distance to four miles per day. He was consistently losing anywhere from one to two pounds per week—which is what we recommend that you do.

Bob early on had convinced Edmond that he should eat more fiber, fruits and vegetables, and cut down on sweets, fats and fried foods. He wasn't actually cutting down much on calories, but was eating more of the right foods. This combination of aerobic exercise and good diet was truly the thing he needed to turn his life around completely. After precisely one year of faithful adherence to his daily regimen, he had practically become a different person in appearance, self-esteem and mental outlook. He had actually lost 80 pounds of ugly fat in one year's time. His energy level and physical condition were the best they had been in years. Those who had seen him infrequently were amazed at his transformation. After that, he went on to become a high-level competitor in racewalking and 1982 Colorado state chairman for the Athletics Congress for that event. The only disadvantage was that he had to junk his entire wardrobe and buy another—a small price to pay, he feels, for his new lifestyle. He embarked on this program in 1980, and is still in trim, athletic condition to this day.

## Recommendations of Nutritional Needs

The U.S. Senate Select Committee on Nutrition and Human Needs has published its dietary recommendations and goals for Americans. These guidelines tell us:

1. You should increase complex carbohydrate consumption by eating more fresh vegetables, fruits and whole grains.
2. You should lower your cholesterol intake by eating fewer eggs, less butter and red meat. Eat more poultry and fish. Substitute low-fat or skim milk for whole milk.
3. You should reduce the total amount of dietary fat and decrease the ratio of saturated to polyunsaturated and monosaturated fats. This can easily be accomplished by avoiding fatty foods and using polyunsaturated fats in their place.
4. You should reduce sugar consumption by approximately 40 percent, eating fewer foods with high sugar content.
5. You should reduce salt intake by reducing the use of table salt and eating fewer processed foods.

The U.S. Department of Agriculture has made the following recommendations in its pamphlet, *Nutrition and Your Health: Dietary Guidelines for Americans.*

> If you need to lose weight, do so gradually. Steady loss of one to two pounds per week until you reach your goal is relatively safe and more likely to be maintained. Long-term success depends upon acquiring new and better habits of eating and exercise. That is why "crash" diets usually fail in the long run.
>
> Do not attempt to lose weight too rapidly. Avoid crash diets that are severely restrictive in the variety of foods they allow. Diets with fewer than 800 calories per day may be hazardous. Some people have developed kidney stones, disturbing psychological changes and other complications while following such diets. A few people have died suddenly and without warning.

If we follow the U.S. guidelines, it means the best way to lose weight is to eat less fat, less red meat and less sugar while increasing fresh vegetables, fresh fruits and whole grains. All you need to do is keep the number of calories consumed lower than what you burn off daily with exercise and normal activities. Avoid dietary excesses and increase exercise.

Dr. Fredric Stare, noted professor at Harvard Medical School, has put forth the following statements about diets and dieting:

1. No one food by itself provides good nutrition. To keep as well nourished as one's genetic potential permits, one must eat a variety of foods from among and within the basic four food groups.
2. Portion size is important and, particularly for meats and dairy products, must be adjusted to caloric (physical) activity, so that desirable weight is reached and maintained.
3. Alcoholic beverages are potent sources of calories. There are indications that alcohol in excess is a carcinogen especially in combination with cigarette smoking.
4. Skipping or skimping on breakfast or lunch and then having a larger dinner is likely to result in intake of more calories in a 24-hour period than having three smaller meals throughout the day.
5. Calories are all alike, whether they come from beef or

bourbon, from sugar or starch or from cheese and crackers. Too many calories are too many calories.

Simply put, if you eat more calories than you burn, you gain; eat less than you burn and you lose! Eat the proper foods and you should never need to deprive yourself of reasonable quantities of food. Exercise and you can increase the amounts of food eaten. Lead that dangerous sedentary life and your food intake must be diminished a lot just to hold the line at your present weight.

## Effects of Food and Drink on Exercise

Food provides energy for internal body processes, muscular activity and body heat. This type of energy comes almost exclusively from carbohydrates and fats. Proteins and vitamins supply essential substances for repair and protection.

There is a common belief that exercise will require you to consume more protein for strength. This is a myth. In fact, too much protein can even be detrimental to strength and endurance during exercise. The muscles need fuel in the form of carbohydrates—not protein—to get the glycogen (the muscles' fuel) to function properly. Excess protein cannot be stored and thus is broken down, causing the release of toxic products such as urea. This urea must be filtered by the blood and excreted by the kidneys. This means the kidneys are doing extra work with excess urination and consequent dehydration. Dehydration and exercise in combination can be dangerous. The result may be decreased performance, constipation, fatigue and even heat stroke in warm weather. Excess protein will also increase blood acidity, with resulting fatigue and irritability. It also increases the loss of calcium and the danger of osteoporosis.

The average-size person, whether an exerciser or not, needs only about 50 grams of protein per day. This requirement can be met with about four average-size servings of any of the following: milk, yogurt, cottage cheese, fish or fowl. In addition there are hidden proteins in breads, cereals, vegetables and fruits. The average person far exceeds his daily protein requirements and, since most protein sources are high in fat, cardiovascular and cancer susceptibility are increased.

Use complex carbohydrates when you wish to increase your energy stores. These complex carbohydrates (breads, cereals, whole grains, pasta and rice, to mention a few) are slow-release fuel sources that give steady and consistent energy to the exerciser. The ideal diet should consist of 60 to 70 percent complex carbohydrates. Although athletes often "load up" on carbohydrates before endurance events, a high-carbohydrate diet as a routine is not a good idea. If the body uses carbohydrates for fuel instead of fat, glycogen supplies run down and an exerciser will run out of energy much faster.

Beware of simple carbohydrates (sugars), since they enter the bloodstream too rapidly, and the resulting speedy increase in blood sugar triggers insulin release to counteract it. Energy levels and exercise endurance then drop rapidly (as much as 25 percent) because of the insulin reaction. The resulting low blood sugar results in marked fatigue and a lessened ability to exercise.

Don't eat a lot of food just before exercising. A full stomach can cause cramping and fatigue. Fats and proteins assimilate very slowly and should be avoided prior to exercise in favor of complex carbohydrates. These provide a constant source of energy without danger of cramping from a full stomach of undigested foods, provided that you wait an hour or two after eating. Practically speaking, an overall balanced diet high in carbohydrates with only moderate or small amounts of fat and protein is best for active people.

There are sport drinks on the market that are supposed to replace electrolytes lost in perspiration. Recent experiments, however, show that water is still the very best replacement fluid available. Most sport drinks, unless very diluted, can actually increase dehydration by impairing the body's ability to absorb water. This is because anything added to water, such as sugar, minerals and electrolytes, slows gastric emptying time, causing the liquid to sit in the stomach instead of entering the bloodstream where it is needed. As you perspire during exercise, the electrolytes, instead of becoming lost, actually become more concentrated and need more water to bring them back into the ideal balance. But don't go overboard and drink too much—excess fluids in the stomach can cause cramping and nausea during exercise. The ADA (American

Dietetic Association) recommends drinking three glasses of water two hours before exercising in hot weather, and another two glasses just before exercise. They recommend drinking plenty of water after exercise to restore water weight loss. This may take many hours during hot weather.

## Become a Label Reader

After choosing the general direction of our diets, we must then start looking at the individual foods that we use in our diets. As a general rule, the less processing that is done to foods the better. Become a label reader so you can know what you are buying. The Food and Drug Administration requires food producers to list ingredients in the diminishing order of their quantity. Take advantage of this information.

"Natural" and "organically grown" are buzz words and powerful sales tools used these days to get people to pay higher prices for foods. They do not necessarily mean anything about the quality of the food you are getting. "Organic" encompasses any chemical compound containing carbon—which means anything grown, animal or vegetable, is organic. So is petroleum, which is derived from animal and vegetable decay and which is the base for most pesticides. "Natural" is another term that is not always what it's cracked up to be. Often "natural" foods can be worse than their well-processed counterparts. Oils used in many natural foods are often coconut and palm oils, which are both very high in saturated fats. Highly saturated fats are known to be a factor in causing cardiovascular and cerebrovascular disease, obesity and various other ailments distressing Americans today. Learn to read between the lines on food packages: "Natural" may be only a modifier of some other word such as "tasting" or "flavor," and graphically placed to mislead you into thinking you are getting something worth spending more for.

When you read "no preservatives" on a label, it is not always a plus. Some preservatives are good, some are bad, some are necessary to prevent premature spoiling and are harmless. Some preservatives such as calcium propionate protect us from the carcinogenic poison aflatoxin in breads and other foods. In addition, it adds calcium to our diet, which we need more of as we get older. The Food and Drug Administration protects us from harmful preservatives in most cases.

Now, let's examine the various components of foods so you can be more knowledgeable about them and so you can wisely select a diet you can live with as you walk your way to fitness.

1. Carbohydrates: Plants represent the main source of carbohydrates in foods. Carbohydrate is one of our most important sources of body energy. Two types of carbohydrates exist in nature: sugars and starches. Grains such as wheat, rice, barley, and oats are rich in starches. Dried beans and potatoes are also starchy and important in everyone's diet. On the other hand, the ordinary table sugar, sucrose, should be avoided. It is loaded with empty calories, is devoid of nutrients and causes unnecessary weight gain and tooth decay. Sugary foods should be avoided in your diet; whole-grain foods and starches should be included. Some doctors advise substituting honey for sugar, but it is not that much superior, nutritionally speaking. It is useful as a flavoring, but many get the mistaken impression that it is not harmful in excess. But it is. It is very wise to reduce your dependence on and taste for sweetness, which is very seductive. Starches are really very low in calories; it is usually the stuff you put on them that causes an overload of calories.

2. Proteins: Meats are our main source of protein, although some protein actually comes from plant sources. When we were growing up, protein was essential to give us the materials to grow on. In later years protein is necessary to replace and revive injured and worn cells and tissues. Adults can get along with surprisingly little protein, but, even so, a minimum must be maintained or deterioration can take place. Since eggs, dairy products and some plants are sources of protein, even vegetarians can get all the protein they need. Americans, by the way, are notorious for overeating proteins, which, as we have pointed out, are poor sources of energy.

3. Fats: The human body requires only about four to six grams of fat a day. Typical Americans eat fifteen to twenty times that amount daily. We should avoid fat as much as possible and reduce our intake of both animal and vegetable

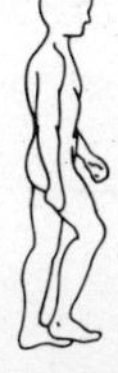

fats. Animal fat adds to the problem of raising blood cholesterol, which can be dangerous because this waxy substance, even though a certain amount is natural in the body, is a major cause of arteriosclerosis, hardening of the arteries, and therefore of heart disease and stroke.

4. Vitamins: There are in nature a series of organic chemicals required by our bodies to keep them functioning properly. These chemicals are needed in very minute quantities and are called vitamins. We should rely on our foods to supply us with these substances. Vitamins are readily available in our natural food sources, such as meats, fish, vegetables, fruits, grains and dairy products. A person who eats a well-balanced diet should have no need for vitamin supplements except in certain circumstances. Some strict vegetarians may be well-advised to take supplementary B vitamins. But millions of dollars are wasted yearly purchasing vitamin supplements that are unnecessary. If you are are a strict vegetarian, or for some reason do not have access to a balanced diet or cannot eat some foods because of a medical problem, then certain vitamin supplements can be of value to make up deficiencies. But most of us should save the money and use it for something else. Taking excess vitamins is usually not harmful to anything except the pocketbook, but vitamins A and D can be toxic in large amounts. The water-soluble vitamins are excreted as waste by the urinary system, but nevertheless may cause such things as kidney stones.

5. Minerals: Vitamins are organic substances needed by the body. Minerals, on the other hand, are inorganic elements required by our system to maintain life and function. These elements include calcium, chloride (salt), potassium, phosphorus, magnesium, sulfur, iron and iodine, among others. These are sufficient in our usual food chain. Some menstruating women require extra iron supplementation.

6. Fiber: Another name for fiber is roughage. Fiber is not a nutrient per se, but is nonetheless vital to our diet and well-being. Roughage increases the bulk of our diet without increasing calories. It is provided by the shells and husks or outer coating of vegetation. Often this valuable portion of vegetable foods has been thrown away. When wheat is ground into flour, the shell or husk of the grain is most often discarded.

The same is true of rice. Whole rice—or brown rice—is shelled and made into white rice. This process increases the caloric content per volume we eat, and discards valuable bulk our systems so badly need.

Now whole-grain cereals, rice and breads are becoming more popular. The person who eats brown rice will get far fewer calories per volume of food ingested than the person who eats white rice, and the food will be better for him. Some grains are as high as 60 percent fiber. To discard this fiber content can significantly increase caloric content per volume eaten.

Not only is whole-grain food lower in caloric content, but because it is less processed, it contains far more of its original vitamin and mineral value. Whole-grain food fiber and roughage aid tremendously in proper digestion. Roughage also absorbs water, fat and sugar in the intestines, binding them and reducing their absorption into the blood, thus helping to keep blood sugar and fat lower, in turn reducing fat deposition. Roughage helps the body maintain regular bowel function and elimination of waste material. The person who eats sufficient fiber will have little or no need for laxatives. In addition, there is growing evidence that high-fiber diets reduce the incidence of diabetes, stroke, heart disease, obesity and colon cancer.

The American Institute for Cancer Research in Washington, D.C., recommends the following guidelines to lower cancer risk:

1. Reduce the intake of dietary fat.
2. Increase the consumption of fiber and roughage in the form of fruits, vegetables and whole-grain cereals.
3. Consume salt-cured, smoked and charcoal-broiled foods only in moderation.
4. Drink alcoholic beverages only in moderation.

Keep these facts in mind when you select your diet. Just as no one can tell you what exercises you will be able to stick with, no one can tell you what diet you will be able to tolerate. You need a realistic diet for your own unique situation.

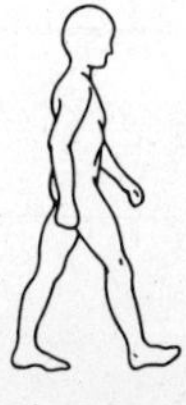

## Start with Gradual Change

Do not alter your diet drastically all at once. Wait at least two weeks into your program until you become hooked on exercise. At first, the changes in exercise habits are enough. Your dietary changes can be spread over time. Also your expectations of losing weight may be too high initially. You might even gain a little. But remember: The weight gain you might experience when you first start to work out is due to toning and building of muscle tissue, which weighs more than the fat you are losing. Even while you might be gaining weight, you will notice your clothes fitting better and your belt coming in a notch or two.

It is interesting that the same diet principles hold true whether you are trying to gain or lose weight. The idea is to get a nutritionally balanced meal that fills your body's caloric needs. If you are trying to lose, you need to reduce your caloric intake by a small amount. If you are trying to gain, the needs are likewise larger by a very few calories.

You will be surprised how few calories make the difference between gain, staying the same, and loss. Reducing 3,500 calories a week off your food consumption will knock off one pound of storage fat. If you are exercising off just 200 calories a day, then you need to cut out only 300 calories a day to lose that pound of fat each week to make the 500. That shouldn't be too tough if you're serious about getting in shape.

Dieting without vigorous exercise can be futile. We humans don't like to consider ourselves part of the animal kingdom, but we are just that. The lower forms of animals can be smarter about what they eat than we humans. The basic biological and physiological rules apply to us as well as animals.

A human being going on a crash diet without exercising is like a hibernating bear! When animals go into hibernation, they have tremendous deposits of storage fat. During hibernation they make few energy demands on this fat, just like us when we are sedentary. During hibernation the animal stops eating—starves, just like us on a fad, restricted diet. The animal's system goes into a conservation phase. Its system says: "It is starvation time again—time to conserve storage fat. Let out only what is absolutely necessary to maintain basic life functions." Thus the animal conserves its fat until spring, surviving the long winter on remarkably little weight loss because Mother Nature has reduced its metabolism to an absolute minimum.

Much the same happens to us when we reduce caloric intake too much, as on a crash diet, and do no additional exercise. Our system senses starvation—hibernation—conservation. Our metabolism is set to a new low. It is truly amazing how low our metabolisms can set themselves during starvation periods. It is part of our natural survival system. People in concentration camps in World War II survived for long periods on extremely few calories per day. Dr. Seiden has seen some obese people cut their calories down to 500 calories per day and hardly lose a pound. We have seen people who have suffered through restrictive diets only to be accused of cheating on those diets by doctors and friends. This tends to make them say, "To hell with it" and give up. Now their system resets the metabolism again, but this time a little lower than before, and the same amount of eating actually made them gain more than they weighed before they began their diet. Does that sound familiar?

That is why many of us have gained back everything—even more than we ever lost on diets—and ended up heavier than when we started. We would have been better off never to have started a diet. How, then, do we avoid this futile and vicious cycle? It is simply done. Start with a couple of weeks of exercise, building yourself up to a rigorous workout level before you even begin to think of dieting. What does that do? It fools your body systems. Activity does just the opposite of what hibernation does. It adjusts your metabolism set-point higher than before. It mobilizes your storage fat to release needed energy.

The body does not need to conserve because it knows you are not hibernating but are very active, and it knows that active animals forage for food when they need it. It does not think it has to conserve to maintain basic life functions. Fat will be metabolized and your extra inches will come off. For a while at first, you will tone and build some muscle so you may even gain—but gain the right kind of pounds, muscle pounds, instead of tearing yourself down through starvation.

## A Little Change Goes a Long Way!

Now when you start our diet, a sensible diet, you will be reducing not more than 500 calories a day from what you have been used to. Cut out fat and sugar calories and your metabolism set-point will remain high because you are going to continue your activity. You will lose unwanted weight permanently, easily and with minimum sacrifice.

The overweight crowd, those more than pleasantly plump, should not find it too difficult to either expend another 500 calories or eat 500 fewer calories. Slow but permanent weight loss is the only viable way to go. If you are trying to gain weight, just eat more nutritionally good foods.

In order to shave 500 calories off your usual diet, make a list of everything you eat over the next few days. Keep the list with you and write down everything as soon as you eat it. Don't wait until the end of the day and expect to remember all things consumed all day. Overeaters have a very convenient amnesia about the snacking done during the day. If you drink coffee and use cream and sugar, those are real calories and they can really mount up. Those little snacks out of vending machines are easily forgotten, but again may add hundreds of unwanted and unneeded calories. Same with the Coke break. Just switching to lo-cal drinks by itself can make a half pound of difference in your weight. Doughnuts and pastries are notoriously high in empty calories. In actuality, 500 calories is just not that much. You might be able to reduce by that much just by eliminating junk foods and substituting them with healthier and more nutritious foods.

When you have written your food intake diary for a couple of days, you will be surprised at all the places you can take away 500 calories without changing most of your eating habits. For instance, one Big Mac by itself is 560 calories and a Burger King Double Beef with Cheese is a whopping 950 calories. You can readily see how eliminating one of these will enable you to attain your goal and then some. In reality, 500 calories will not be missed.

Here are a few calorie-reducing hints:

1. Drink coffee or tea without sugar or cream.

2. Avoid the normal soft drinks and change to tea, skim milk or unsweetened fruit or vegetable juices. Of course you can substitute the best drink of all—cool, clear water, preferably distilled.

3. If you eat sandwiches for lunch, make them open-face, and reduce or eliminate butter, margarine, ketchup or mayonnaise. If you must use a spread, use a vegetable margarine that is cholesterol free.

4. If you eat meat, reduce the quantity and eat it only once a day. Eat more poultry (without the skin) and fish than beef to keep the fat calories lower. If you must eat beef, it is grades such as "U.S. Good" or "Choice" that are lower in fat and thus healthier for you.

5. Try to get into the habit of making your lunch just soup and salad. That is all you need to keep your energy levels up.

6. Don't eat Danish or doughnuts for breakfast or at a coffee break—substitute whole-grain toast or a muffin. Coffee breaks at the office are often an empty calorie disaster. Bring a nutritious snack to work instead.

7. Try to replace sweets and fried snacks (like potato chips) with raw vegetables and fruits.

8. If you reduce the quantity you eat at meals by only 20 percent you will probably drop 500 calories a day without changing any of your bad eating habits. But if you're smart you'll eat less junk food, more good food, fill your tummy so it is comfortable and happy, and you will LOSE WEIGHT at a rate of up to a pound a week.

The key is to reduce gradually—not more than one to two pounds a week. If you lose more, the body will sense a starvation mode and will slow the metabolism as we have warned. All the effort that you can muster in planning a healthy and nutritious diet will pay back dividends many times over. The combination of the correct diet and correct exercise will make the rest of your life a vigorous and healthy one. But in addition to these you must also eliminate any bad habits that can either derail or slow your progress drastically. And be sure to keep walking every day!

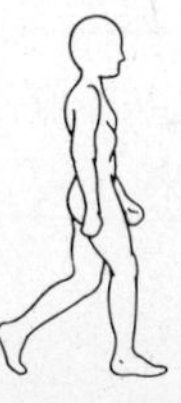

## CHAPTER 10

# FIGHT KILLER HABITS

*"No matter how far you have gone on a wrong road, turn back."*
—old Turkish proverb

---

If you don't drink too much, smoke tobacco, do drugs or lean on tranquilizers as a constant crutch, you can probably skip this chapter. Otherwise try to read it with an open mind and think seriously about its contents so that you can help others. In this book we are asking you to make a lifestyle change. It makes little sense to develop a whole set of HEALTHY habits while maintaining others that work to shorten life and injure you. If you are a slave to any of these killer habits, now is the time to turn your addiction around.

Realize that one of the biggest problems (as when you are overweight or out of shape) is denial! Seldom will you find any addict who will admit to his addiction until it is too late to save him from his personal hell on earth. If you have a drinking problem, smoke, mess around with pot and other drugs, or rely heavily on tranquilizers—you probably are an addict. "Sure I smoke," you say to yourself, "but I'm not an addict." But in fact that's just what you are! Smoking is among the strongest of addictions, rivaling even heroin. That is why it is so tough to quit. You need all the help and encouragement you can get to stop any addictive habit. (Read Chapter 15 on working with your health professional.)

Let's look at the killer habits one by one.

## Smoking

Smoking, a true curse on mankind, is a true addiction. Anyone who denies this is a member of the tobacco industry or is just plain ignorant of the facts. If you do smoke, the best way to quit is to go "cold turkey," as many have successfully done. It can be very hard to do but is more effective than tapering off, which allows for too much backsliding. However you do it, whether by joining a class under professional guidance or suffering through withdrawal pangs independently, it absolutely must be done as soon as possible. If four fully loaded 747 airliners crashed in the USA every single day killing all aboard, can you imagine the uproar that something be done about it? Yet that is precisely the toll that cigarette smoking is taking on the citizens of our country. Find some way to quit—try every way you can until you are successful. Millions have had success, so why not you? Why should you quit? Let us count the whys:

1. You are a fool if you don't. The evidence against it is now overwhelming. Research clearly shows that smokers have a much higher risk of heart disease and heart attacks, strokes, kidney disease, lung disease, hardening of the arteries, high blood pressure, cancer, colds, lost days from work, infections, skin and complexion problems, allergies, circulatory defects, miscarriages and offspring with birth defects. In addition, your skin wrinkles prematurely making you look older than your true age, and you smell horrible! You are rapidly becoming a "leper" in our enlightened society. Estimates say that each cigarette, or "coffin nail," as they were called sixty years ago, shortens your breathing-impaired life by about three minutes. If you cannot stop this disgusting habit then it may not be worth your time to try to get into physical shape. The two things are too antagonistic.
2. If you don't worry about your own future, think about your loved ones—your spouse and children. Now definitive

studies (that evil empire the Tobacco Institute notwithstanding) show that secondhand smoke is very detrimental to those around you, because the smoke that has not deposited most of its poisons in your lungs is available to others. The Environmental Protection Agency has made available some startling facts:

a. Up to 5,000 non-smoking Americans will die this year of lung cancer caused by exposure to secondhand smoke from a smoking family member or working companion.

b. Researchers have found the blood carbon monoxide levels in non-smokers double when they sit among smokers, even in a well-ventilated room.

c. It will take several hours for the blood levels to return to normal after a non-smoker leaves a room that contained a smoker.

d. Children's lungs will not grow as rapidly as normal when exposed to secondhand smoke.

e. A non-smoker in a smoke-filled room for an hour will inhale as much cancer-causing material as a smoker will inhale from more than five cigarettes.

Cigarettes kill 350,000 people per year in the U.S. Even so, billboards, magazines and newspapers continue to sell lung destruction, cancer, emphysema and heart disease to the American public with their irresponsible advertising of the deadly and noxious product, mostly directed toward the young to get them hooked. We must combat the scourge of tobacco through legislation and boycotts in future years.

We could go on and on explaining the horrors of this disgusting habit, but you are no doubt getting the drift that we do not like this legal product one bit. How do you think the Food and Drug Administration would rate tobacco if it were a new product just about to enter the market? Do you think it could actually be tested thoroughly and be passed on to the public as a harmless and beneficial product for society?

Less than 28 percent of the total population now smokes, and the American Medical Association is doing its utmost to cut it even further by attempting to make it as extinct as a dodo bird by the time the year 2000 rolls around. But tobacco lobbies are powerful and rich, and it will be quite a job to accomplish this. By promoting smokeless cigarettes, so that addicts can get their poisonous nicotine fix by sucking warmed air over unburned tobacco, the tobacco industry will go to any means to continue selling its deadly product. If you are addicted, it will take more than words from us to persuade you to quit. It must come from a powerful inner urge and conviction.

We contend that the better aerobic shape you are in, the less likely you are to smoke. Aerobic conditioning and cigarette smoking are absolutely incompatible, the glamorous cigarette ads notwithstanding. If you take up brisk walking and discover the joys of breathing freely, you will not want to compromise this great feeling by inhaling noxious smoke into your lungs.

## Alcohol

Alcoholism is the number-one drug problem in the world today. At least one in 10 and maybe even more people in the USA are alcoholics or potential alcoholics. Alcohol is three times more of a problem than all the "hard drugs" put together at this time. If you drink more than three alcoholic drinks daily to pull yourself through, you probably are on the verge of being addicted or already are addicted. See if you can quit for a few days, and if you can't, seek professional help. Here are a few facts that you should know:

1. About half of alcoholics are women.
2. Only about 3 percent of "alkies" are skid-row bums. Alcoholism ranges through all the social classes; there is no group that is exempt.
3. It is a physical disease, a drug addiction, in part genetic, and is treatable.
4. Denial is the most important factor keeping an alcoholic from overcoming a drinking problem. Closet drinkers abound and you are only fooling yourself if you think it is making you operate more efficiently. You can be destroying yourself and your loved ones if it goes on and on. Cirrhosis of the liver, brain damage and serious accidents are common results.

Alcoholism has for some time been classed as a disease instead of a moral problem. This disease takes its toll on both the body and the psyche. Cure is extremely difficult, but exercise can be of great help in lessening its effects. One study showed that 20 alcoholics who walked or jogged at least a mile a day showed a great improvement in self-esteem, sleep patterns and physical fitness as compared to non-exercisers who showed no changes. Among 18 men hospitalized for psychiatric problems, including alcoholism, daily bouts of exercise for three weeks increased fitness, decreased hypochondria and shortened some of their hospital stays.

Walking helps recovering alcoholics physically by improving metabolism and speeding detoxification, and psychologically by improving self-esteem, sense of well-being and mastery over the disease as a part of their treatment. Some Alcoholics Anonymous groups have patients walk or jog at a moderate pace for three or four miles four or more times per week before the regular AA meeting. Invariably the exercisers are more relaxed at the meetings than the non-exercisers. Morning runs or walks allow recovering alcoholics to launch the day with positive activity that provides a sense of achievement and reinforces the commitment to abstinence.

Here is a true story of a 44-year-old alcoholic who used walking and jogging to overcome his disease. He says, "What has this exercise program done for me? I've gone from 152 to 137 pounds, and at 5' 81/2" that is pretty trim. My blood pressure is down to a normal 120/80 and my heart rate at rest is 56 to 60. My waistline went from 32 inches to 29. I sleep like a log and need less sleep to function at peak efficiency in my job. Mentally, I'm more alert and less tense. I have a happier outlook. I can control my temper better and enjoy working with people. I have found a way to unwind without the help of John Barleycorn. Not all these improvements have been the result of just a good exercise program, but it certainly played an important part, and I hate to think where I'd be without it. I'm not proud of my alcoholism—but I am proud of what I've done about it. And grateful. Boy, it's nice to feel good again."

## Hard Drugs

Hard drugs have been a thorn in the side of civilization through recorded history. Those in the drug culture always have denied that they had a problem or that their habit was really hurting them or anyone else. These so-called "recreational drugs" will ultimately destroy the user who doesn't quit or seek help. If you are smoking pot or using cocaine with the idea that it is not dangerous, and is even helping you, you are already at a point in your habit where irrationality prevents you from making responsible decisions. Again, as with alcohol or cigarettes, if you are addicted, it will take powerful means to correct the situation by means of a personal commitment, or through a professional counselor.

## Tranquilizers

One of the growing tragedies of today's society is our reliance on prescription drugs. Tranquilizers and anti-depressants and other mind-altering drugs are being abused at an epidemic rate. Careless or incompetent doctors are a part of the problem. Another contributing factor is a patient's scheme to get more of these than the physician ever intended with the idea that if a little is good then a lot must be real good. Some people go to more than one doctor without telling the others, just to get the extra drugs. If your doctor has you on a mind-altering drug for more than a few weeks and isn't monitoring you to get you off the medication as soon as possible, you must get a second opinion. If you are getting these drugs illegally because you cannot get along without them, then you are just as much a junkie as those on hard drugs.

Again, we don't expect many drug abusers to read this book, but if you have a loved one or good friend who needs help, we hope we have put the problems in perspective and motivated you to help them seek guidance and confront themselves with their problem.

## Change Before It's Too Late

Don't fall for that old cliché, "You can't teach an old dog new tricks." Anyone who is incapable of making personal changes in his life is in deep trouble. It won't be easy, but with enough motivation it may not be as hard as you think. If you say "I just can't," it really means, "I just don't want to even try." There is no habit that is impossible to break. All of them we have mentioned in this book are being broken every day by truly motivated people.

Long-term habits may become so ingrained they are viewed as necessities. This is also true of walking, but in a positive sense. The bad habits are breakable, so break them—cold turkey. Many think that they need drugs or alcohol or cigarettes to calm themselves down or to escape reality or to relieve everyday stresses. We will demonstrate to you in Chapter 11 that walking is just as good a stress reliever as potent life-destroying drugs with good instead of dangerous side effects. Get help and support if necessary, but break these habits now before it is too late.

**CHAPTER 11**

# STRESS

*"Often a voluntary change of activity is as good or better than rest—for example, when either fatigue or enforced interruption prevents us from solving a mathematical problem, it is better to go for a walk than simply to sit around. Substituting demands on our musculature for those previously made on the intellect not only gives our brain a rest but helps us avoid worrying about frustrating interruption. Stress on one system helps to relax another."*

—Hans Selye, M.D.,
Author of *Stress Without Distress*

---

Everyone lives with stress of varying degrees—the surprising fact is that a certain amount is necessary and even desirable. It motivates us, helps us get things done, makes us bring about changes in our lives and improves our lot. Was it stress about personal health that prompted you to buy this book? If that stress is strong enough, you will do something about your situation. When stress brings about action it is usually good. If it merely causes you to worry, it can be harmful. Negative stress can destroy your health. Stress that cannot be reduced by action will also destroy your health. The real trick is to turn stress into your ally—a motivation for stress-reducing action.

Too much stress of the wrong kind, if not relieved, can be a potent destroyer of health. It can make gastric juices squirt in the stomach when they are supposed to be quiet; it boosts blood pressure, leading to strokes and heart attacks; it pushes people to drug abuse and alcoholism. Stress-related failings ruin marriages, friendships and jobs. Stress leads to fights and accidents; it makes lives unpleasant—and shorter. Read on and you will see how you can literally walk away from your stressful situations.

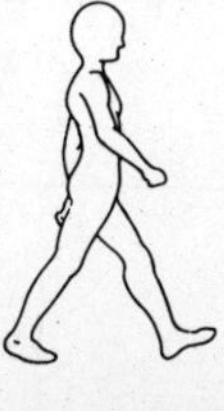

## Be Prepared to Cope

Emotional stress, the fight or flight reflex, has been with us since man showed up on earth. The caveman could either stand and fight if he chose, or run like the dickens to get away from danger. In times of stress or danger, the body's powerful chemical, adrenaline, flows, making us alert and strong so we can address the impending emergency. Have you ever narrowly escaped a serious automobile accident? At the time, it is all instinct. Your body is numb, concentrated on reacting to the situation. Then, when the danger is past, you feel your heart pounding very hard, your mouth turning to "cotton," and your tongue thickening. Your pulse is rapid, and you feel as though you are on an elevator that is dropping too suddenly. Only afterward are you truly aware of the great stress that was put on your body and mind. A weak, underexercised heart can literally be frightened to death in emergency situations.

But what happens, as is so often the case in modern society, if we can neither fight nor flee an impending disaster or emergency? All the unreleased stress can build up within the body to dangerous levels, levels which an unfit body may not be able to withstand. When an impending disaster, real or imagined, occurs, your body responds automatically. You don't have to think "Do something!" Your brain automatically alerts the appropriate hormones to disperse immediately. Your heart rate rises, pumping more blood to the muscles; your lungs provide more oxygen; and sugar and fat reserves are released. Every time stress is applied, your body mobilizes for fight or flight. You have used extra energy uncontrollably. Disaster often occurs when your energy-producing potential is too low—when you are physically unfit to cope.

## An Up-and-Down Effect

Undue stress can have a detrimental effect on the body. Taking a simple analogy, think of the constant fluctuations of the stock market. The sympathetic and parasympathetic nervous systems in your body work in a similar fashion. Your nervous system has an accelerating chemical (sympathin). It helps you cope with tense situations like confronting a growling dog or assailant, going out and finding your car won't start when you need to go some place in a hurry, or any other crisis, either genuine or imagined. When the crisis is over, the body slows you down rapidly with an opposing chemical (acetycholine). Stock-market inconsistencies are natural; however, such an up-and-down effect on your body takes its toll. You can swamp your sympathetic nerve endings with a flood of the body's own powerful chemicals, and this is obviously a stress on your system in its own right.

Now some astute psychologists and psychiatrists are realizing that physical exercise is the best and most practical means to relieve many of the worries and stresses that are inevitably an integral part of modern-day life. Valium and other tranquilizers, nevertheless, are still some of the most overprescribed drugs in the United States. Drug dependency is one of the real tragedies of contemporary society. We must get the message across to everyone that action absorbs anxiety in a much safer fashion than drugs. It is now known that human bodies actually produce their own natural tranquilizers, known as endorphins, which are released into the bloodstream after a certain amount of exercise—a minimum of more than 20 minutes of brisk, continuous, rhythmic movement, which is characteristic of brisk walking.

## A Diversionary Tactic

It is an unfortunate fact that people who have not experienced the joys and positive effects of walking tend to discount it as a valid and beneficial exercise. Most people think that mere diversions such as watching television, playing bridge or checkers, or having a social drink is enough to forget your troubles for awhile. But none of these diversions gives the immediate antidote to stress that a good walk will, because none has any aerobic value. Besides, a good walk with someone else is a better diversion because it is aerobic in nature, very sociable, a good morale builder and mood enhancer. It's easy to take regular walks once you get started, and easier yet when you have someone to take them with.

Dr. Paul Dudley White, who was one of our country's most renowned and respected cardiologists and deemed dean emeritus of personal fitness, said that a brisk five-mile walk will do more good for an overstressed and unhappy but otherwise healthy adult than all the medicine and psychology in the world. Dr. White was also quoted as saying, "A half-hour or more of fast walking every day is very necessary for one's optimal health including that of the brain. The body and the mind are not separate entities." The part of the brain that controls the walking movement is called the motor cortex. It is extremely close to the part of the brain strata that deals with thought, feeling and association processes. Since we must use the motor cortex during the walking movement, the closeness of the two functions creates a parallel effect on thinking and feeling, according to some researchers. Regular aerobic physical exercise has been proven time and time again to greatly decrease the effects of stressful situations. Worries just evaporate after a certain amount of the activity; calmness and a sense of well-being prevail.

## Sound Body, Sound Mind

As the ancient Greeks understood so well more than 2,500 years ago, the mind and body cannot really be separated. They espoused the idea that a sound mind and sound body are intertwined into a healthy whole. Train your body and you are on the road to training your mind and your psyche. Developing "nerves of steel" is a part of becoming fit. You must build the equipment you need to cope with stress. Medical science measures total fitness in the terms of one's ability to tolerate stresses, which constitute many of the struggles of life. You may consider stress to be your enemy. This is not necessarily so. In reality, your true enemy is unfitness. Stress, on the other hand, is not particular—it can become your ally or your enemy's ally. It inevitably joins the stronger of the two. If you are truly in good physical shape, stress will be on your side; but if you are unfit, you've got real trouble with the stress and the unfitness compounding each other in a vicious downward spiral to poorer health, and possibly even to your demise.

Dr. White also noted that the power failure and transit strikes in Manhattan in the mid-1960s, which were extremely stress-producing and traumatic for most New Yorkers, actually had great beneficial side effects. The two events forced thousands and thousands of people to walk to places that they would never have dreamed of walking to otherwise—some strolling 10 or 15 miles across the bridges to their homes in other parts of the Big Apple. He said that these events got more people to realize the joys of walking by doing it than he and his colleagues had been able to do in the previous 15 or 20 years. Many of these New Yorkers continued to walk more and more as a matter of preference because they suddenly started feeling better, calmer, less "stressed out" because of the exercise.

## Breakdowns Can Be Avoided

Dr. Hans Selye, who devoted more than 40 years of his life researching the effects of stress mechanisms and became the world's leading authority on the subject, postulated that each of us possesses at birth a given amount of what he called "adaptational energy." When that energy is used up, we experience a mental or physical breakdown. One way to avoid such a breakdown is by deliberately directing stress at varying body systems. This can best be done by getting into the total body exercise that brisk walking affords.

In a well-known experiment to demonstrate the beneficial effects of exercise, Dr. Selye put 10 sedentary rats in a cage with blinding lights, very loud noises and irregular electric shocks to create a very stressful situation for them. They all died in less than a month from this psychological trauma. He then put 10 rats on an exercise program, on a treadmill, until they were in very good physical condition. After subjecting these rats to the exact same conditions for a month, they were all well and actually thriving. The sedentary rats did not have the strength to withstand the psychological stresses that the conditioned rats handled easily. He had demonstrated that muscular systems and physical conditioning have a significant effect upon how stresses can be handled.

The average contemporary American is very sedentary yet overstimulated. Stresses of all kinds are present in everyday life; there is little chance of relief unless we confront them in an active way. All of us have personal problems that cause tension. Actually it is not the problems themselves, but how we view and address them that are important. It can either "get to us" or we can take positive action against it and get relief. A certain amount of stress in our lives is necessary and even desirable. There is helpful stress called "eustress" and harmful stress called "distress." Dr. Selye once said, "Stress is the spice of life; the absence of it is death." Without any stress at all, life would be very bland and uninteresting.

## Balancing the Effects of Stress

Often people become so accustomed to stress that they become unaware of it; nevertheless, they can suffer the debilitating effects without feeling undue tenseness. It does not affect only those with high-pressure lives—many underachievers experience the worry of leading unfulfilled lives, or of not being what they would like to be. Often it is not events that cause stress but the personal views we take of those events. One person may thrive on a stress that may be perceived as devastating to another. The stronger and more vigorous we are, the more we can fend off the debilitating effects of stressful situations. You need not be enslaved—you can survive by managing stress rather than having it devastate you.

Dr. Clinton Weiman, medical director of Citibank, one of the world's largest banks, found that employees had fewer problems with high blood pressure, excess weight, chronic fatigue and other disabilities if they worked under an optimum amount of stress. He found that either too much or too little was associated with more disease. The fact is that either of these conditions could be corrected with a sensible walking program. Suppose you work at a desk job and you come home washed out, your energy completely gone. You dread the thought of exercising—yet the minute you start you begin to feel better. By the end of 30 minutes you are restored. You may have felt tired, but you find to your surprise that you weren't tired at all—just oxygen depleted. It is a pleasant discovery to make indeed!

## Take Some Easy Days

There will inevitably be some days when you just don't want to exercise too hard. The thought of pushing too hard will leave you cold and unreceptive. On those days, don't despair. Take a slow walk—a walk for your mentality, to enjoy nature or your thoughts. Not only can walking do a lot for you physically, it can also do some wonders for the mind as well. It can help you:

- Solve your problems,
- Reduce mental as well as physical stress,
- Increase your creative thoughts,
- Overcome depressions and anxieties,
- Boost your memory power.

These benefits will occur even during vigorous workouts, but you don't need to go full tilt every day, and it is probably better if you don't. Easy walking days will still burn off the calories, though the aerobic gains will be less with the slower pace. But don't worry about that. Just walk away from your problems at your most comfortable aerobic pace.

As you walk along you can find yourself daydreaming. Even on the most scenic and interesting walks your mind can begin to take wing and fantasize. If you walk the same route all the time, sheer boredom will trigger the process of daydreaming. Did you ever get caught daydreaming as a kid and get chided for it by your teacher or parent? That was their mistake. Recently a lot has been discovered about daydreams and fantasy. It is in reality a high-powered mental activity—a powerful problem-solving activity. The trick is to harness it, and your walks can help you do that.

## Walking Stimulates Right-Brain Activity

While daydreaming, you are using the creative half of your brain, the right side. The left half is mostly devoted to logical or mathematical-type thinking. According to John G. Young, M.D., psychiatric consultant and author of *SELECT: Creative Innovative Approaches*, recent developments show that the difference between the two halves of the brain is not as dramatic as previously thought, but it is still true to some degree. Often when faced with a perplexing problem, you put the left side of the brain to work. But maybe simple logic doesn't do the trick and you draw a total blank. You give up. You try to put it on hold by looking for some diversion, by doing something else. But in reality you are not getting it out of your

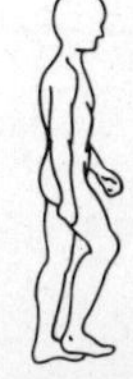

mind at all. The right side of the brain is still working on the problem subconsciously. It works differently, ignoring logic as it works. It does not use the "proper" steps of problem solving. It works in mysterious and unorthodox ways—and very often succeeds. You may think that brilliant ideas come right out of the blue, but in reality they come from the subconscious in the right half of your brain.

Why do we mention all this? Because when you walk and let your mind wander and get into that semi-dreamlike state, the creative part of your brain takes over. The more you daydream, wonder or let your thoughts fly or go unbridled, the quicker and deeper you go into creative thinking. Whenever you have a knotty problem that is getting the best of you, do what Chief Justice William O. Douglas and Albert Einstein used to do—go out for a lengthy walk. That walk will help you find a solution quicker than almost anything else you can do.

## Walking Keeps Your Memory Fit

Walk for a better memory. Reducing the circulation of blood flow and oxygen to the brain is a major cause of memory difficulties. Any activity that improves your cardiovascular and pulmonary systems as walking does is going to help your thinking and memory alike. Any activity that promotes creative thought, problem solving and any other mental activity will also help maintain an active memory. Memory is greatly dependent on mental relationships and is stimulated by other thoughts; we are reminded of things by similar or related concepts or objects. Keep exercising your mind as well as your body and the dividends can be enormous. Walking will allow you to do this more easily by thoroughly oxygenating your brain, and you will worry less about stressful circumstances.

In addition to walking, keep your mind active by reading, taking adult education courses, strolling through museums and galleries, traveling, attending concerts and plays and the like. Lead an active life. Exercise your mind as much as you do your body. Don't be afraid to challenge your mind to its limits.

## Mix Your Mental and Fitness Walks

Make it a point to smell the roses on your daily walks. Start trying to stay alive and take the time to be human as humans were designed to be. Find relaxation in your walking activity, moving in a manner that is not only sensuous and natural but calculated, paced and controlled. Movement is strong medicine. Bringing your body to maximum efficiency will free your mind and emotions to do their best. You will find yourself living more comfortably and calmly as you walk away from the stresses and anxieties that we all have.

Walk to be creative. Sadly, most of our formal schooling in our formative years is aimed at logistics, mathematics, rote memory and such, but not creativity. Creativity is really nothing more than a specialized form of problem solving. Creativity is problem solving that fills needs. To be creative you must use imagination, mental imagery, flights of fancy, daydreams. Walking can help you do that. There is nothing new about this idea. Albert Einstein readily admitted his greatest accomplishments came about while daydreaming, and that long walks were among his greatest allies in bringing about these immensely productive musings. He came onto the theory of relativity while walking along a hillside looking at the changing cloud formations. Others have had similar experiences. Most Nobel Prize winners will tell you that their greatest accomplishments came about while they were daydreaming or during periods of free-floating imagination.

Think about your problems and achievements. How often have you found solutions and bright ideas while lost in reverie? How often have you awakened from a dream you could hardly remember, but with the answer to a problem that had been hounding you? Walking will help you spend more time in your creative mode of thinking because of its relaxing qualities. It just happens that way—believe us!

## Make Your Walks Interesting

Now that we have convinced you why you should take mental walks, we will give you some ideas on where to take them. The choice is only limited by our imaginations. How about your own neighborhood? We drive around and through it almost daily, yet there are always things that we haven't noticed before if we walk through it. Get out and enjoy looking at distinctive features of houses and yards. You might even meet some nice neighbors as you walk along. Visit an old neighborhood where you have lived in the past. Nostalgia and pleasant memories make it fun to reminisce about old times.

Cemeteries are great places to walk. They are park-like and the residents won't bother you at all with boisterous activity. There is very little traffic and it is a quiet and respectful place to walk. You can learn a lot of history by noting what is on all the old gravestones and monuments. You will often see beautiful old trees and perhaps some animal wildlife.

Go to the local zoo. The zoo isn't just for kids—it is for kids at heart as well, and that should include all of us. A trip there will add a great deal of enjoyment to your walk and make you forget your cares as you watch the animals.

Stroll though nearby parks, forests. foothills and mountains, around local lakes, historic districts, seashores—take advantage of the natural wonders that are nearby. Or visit local museums and galleries. You won't get your heart rate up, but remember that this is a walk for the mind as well as the legs. There is so much to learn in this world and so little time to do it. Make it fun and interesting.

Shopping malls are good places to walk when the weather outside is something less than pleasant. More and more malls are opening up for walkers two hours or more before the stores open. This is of mutual advantage for the walkers and store owners for obvious reasons. Window shopping can be fun, but if you are the impulsive type, leave your credit cards safely at home.

Campuses have a nice atmosphere for walking. The educational environment is often stimulating, and you might enjoy this mental walk so much that you will get the inspiration to further your learning.

There is no end to places where we can take our mental walks. We can always use the imagination granted to us, by getting our brains oxygenated from walking, to discover new and exciting places to explore. The main thing is to get out and do it for our bodies and minds—to alleviate stresses and everything else that might be temporarily bothering us.

CHAPTER 12

# WALKING AND SEX

*"When you are out there using your body in a very basic way, looking your best, feeling your best, and knowing you're getting even better, that's attractive. Let's face it: good health and its pursuit is always sexually attractive."*

—William Finley and Marion Weinstein,
Authors of *Racewalking*

---

We knew we could get your attention!

What does sex have to do with walking? Now that we have devoted quite a bit of space to bad habits, let us dwell on a good one. Sex is one of our strongest motivators, so let's use it to our advantage. It is also one of the least understood aspects of life in general, so let's clear up misunderstandings.

If you are now starting into the middle years of your life, don't feel that you have nothing to look forward to. There is plenty of spice in the life ahead—better spice than you might imagine. A person who keeps fit can remain sexually active to the last day of life regardless of age—and many do just that. One of the greatest retardants to sexuality in advanced years is poor circulation. Keep fit with a vigorous walking program and follow good health habits like those we describe here, and that vigor will translate into all aspects of your life—sex included.

In *The Aerobics Program for Total Well-Being*, Kenneth Cooper, M.D., wrote about conditioning and sex: "This is a subject for which quantifiable data are lacking, yet there does seem to be a positive relationship between aerobic conditioning and a satisfying sex life. Many times over the past twenty years, I have had patients volunteer the information that their sex lives have improved in response to regular physical exercise, and when both partners are involved, this relationship seems to be enhanced even more."

Your sexual prowess when you are 80 or older may well depend on how you take care of yourself today and in the future. That is a mighty powerful motivation to get out and walk every day of the year, whether you are young, middle-aged or a Gray Panther. Good, active sex in your later years can certainly add a lot to that quality of life we talked about in the beginning of this book. If you think it won't be important to you, consider your spouse. A sexually inactive partner can be extremely frustrating to the healthier half of the couple. Don't let your spouse or lover down!

A walking program like the one we recommend in this book will give your sex life a real boost. You'll look and feel better and improve how you feel about yourself. You'll notice most of your muscles becoming firmer, your belly flattening, hips, thighs and buttocks shaping up, and you will be achieving a generally healthy overall appearance—a great turn-on for both partners. If you feel all out of shape, sloppy, fat and unappealing to others, however, it will be readily apparent to all, and any semblance of sensuality will be lost. You must feel good about yourself before others can do likewise.

We think of good sex as a strength and endurance event—in order to have both quality and quantity you must have both energy and sensuality. If you have not built up strength and a robust nature, if you're always fatigued and feel flabby, you will respond accordingly—much to the disappointment of your partner. Sex raises your blood pressure and heart rate just as brisk walking does. Your nervous and cardiovascular systems are important parts of a vigorous sex act. Some positions can cause muscular fatigue unless you are in shape. If you need to stop and catch your breath in the middle of making love, the all-important timing and much of the magic of the moment will be lost. The best thing to do is to get into shape and stay there for the rest of your life through healthwalking.

If you women readers have to nag your partner to keep up this health program, it will be well worth it to you. Remember that in our society women outlive men by considerable years. Your nagging now can keep your bed and breakfast partner alive and functioning to his full potential. There need not be all those lonely years of widowhood in our society. Think of the exercise-walking program as investing in a sort of sexual IRA account for both partners, so that you can reap the benefits in later years.

But sex isn't important to you only for the pleasure it will bring to your future years—it is important to your general mental and physical health. There is evidence that men who have an active sex life are less likely to develop prostate disease, which can lead to severe urogenital problems and surgery. Sex is a strong stress reducer and can help to keep your blood pressure within normal ranges. Sexually active people tend to keep themselves more involved, mentally alert and progressive in their attitudes toward the world and life in general. It is vital to keep a young attitude as you grow older chronologically, and nothing can keep your attitude youthful better than a healthy, active sex life.

Show us someone who has lost interest in sex and we'll show you someone who probably has also lost interest in work, friends and many of the other things that make life enjoyable. Good sex is a natural antidepressant, and evidence shows it also gives a natural analgesic pain relief. It is too bad that more is not done to encourage this aspect of our lifestyles.

As for motivation, too many people, once they take sex off their high-priority list, seem to give up on many other beneficial considerations; for example, they lose interest in their appearance. Attracting a sexual partner is still one of the main reasons to look good. Sex motivates us to perform well in all aspects of our life—professional, social, educational, athletic, personal—you name it. It is therefore important that we keep this powerful motivating force alive and healthy. To do this:

1. Walk vigorously and aerobically for 45 minutes or longer every day.
2. Eat the proper healthy foods, but not in excess of daily needs.
3. Avoid excessive alcohol and all tobacco products.
4. Avoid all illicit and prescription drugs that are not absolutely necessary to your well-being.

If you happen to have a sexual dysfunction now, do not assume that it is for life. Impotence is rather common and can usually be treated effectively or cured. A healthy sex life is very important to the quality of your future life. Seek the help of a doctor or sex therapist to solve your problem as soon as possible. If your doctor tells you that at your age sex isn't important, don't believe a word he says and go talk to someone else who is more knowledgeable about sex. Then read Chapter 15 and go about finding yourself another doctor.

For that sexy, youthful appearance with a minimum of wrinkles, you cannot beat vigorous aerobic exercise. It is useful in either ironing wrinkles out or preventing them in the first place. It has been found that what makes the face red—oxygen—makes it rugged as well. Also, it is now well-documented that cigarette smoking, the archenemy of aerobic exercise, often causes premature wrinkling of the skin. Some doctors in Finland took skin samples from the arms of 29 middle-aged, active men and compared them with similar samples from 29 middle-aged sedentaries. It was found that the skin of the heavy exercisers was thicker, stronger and more elastic than the skin of their less active peers. The researchers explained the results suggest the skin reflects an adaptation to habitual endurance training by increasing its mass and strengthening its structure. Who can deny that a great complexion and fine skin tone over the entire body is a sexual turn-on?

The editors of *PREVENTION* magazine health books wrote in *Future Youth: How to Reverse the Aging Process:* "According to Art Mollen, D.O., founder of the Southwest Health Institute in Phoenix, Arizona, and author of *The Mollen Method*, a study of fit men showed that they had more sexual desire and a better attitude about sex than men who were out of shape. What's more, the study found that physically active men in their late forties and fifties had sex as frequently as the younger men in the study. In fact, the author of the study, Lawrence Katzman, Ph.D., believes that exercise is the best prescription for problems like impotence, lack of desire, premature ejaculation, or the inability to achieve orgasms."

You women of 50 or older who have suffered the demise of your mate or a different kind of separation face a perplexing problem. There just aren't that many good elderly men left from which to choose. Those who are available are too often looking for a nurse rather than a mate. They have not been walking away from old age. Here's something to ponder—if the men your own age and older can't pass muster or just aren't available, then get yourself in the best possible shape and compete for the younger guys. There is no reason why you should limit your social contacts to men your age or older. If your health habits make you physically and philosophically 10 years younger than your chronological age, then broaden your range of social contacts to those several years your junior. That will open a lot of doors and possibilities for you, thus rewarding you for taking care of yourself.

There is one thing that we cannot fully understand. Why is the heart always the symbol of love? It is admittedly the one-pound pump that circulates the life-giving oxygenated blood to all parts of the body. But clearly, the brain and its thought processes are the computer that governs all the body's processes, including the sex glands. When you think of your loved one, it is not your heart getting you excited, but your "headquarters," the brain. Our theory is that most of the writers and lyricists throughout history would have been very hesitant about calling lovers "sweetbrains" instead of sweethearts, thus cramping their romantic flourishes.

## CHAPTER 13

# OVERCOMING DISABILITIES

*"The average man becomes physiologically old early in life, which may explain how many succumb to disease of chronic deterioration at an early age."*

—John Naughton, M.D.

---

Even after reading all the good stuff about the beneficial effects of walking, you may still be worried about undertaking a walking program because of a special and troublesome ailment that has caused you to become a sedentary couch potato. In the past, doctors advised victims of heart disease, arthritis, obesity, emphysema and diabetes to diet and take it easy on the physical exercise. Fortunately, most knowledgeable and informed physicians have changed their tune these days. If your physician has not encouraged you to increase your physical activity, do the following: Ask him for a satisfactory reason why he feels you should not exercise. How will it harm you? If you can't exercise, what *can* you do to get into better physical condition? Then go get a second opinion.

The point is, very few medical conditions are not improved by bettering the general condition of the entire body. Your doctor or other health professional may have a very good reason to limit your activity out of concern for possibly aggravating an existing condition, but you have every right to know why and whether there is anything you can do to change your lot. We will now address some of the disabilities that afflict us in modern-day society on which walking has a beneficial effect.

## Heart Disease

When Dr. Seiden was in medical school, the fledgling doctors were taught that whenever anyone had a heart attack, he should be put to bed for six to eight weeks while the heart healed. This unfortunate soul should then be trained to lead a sedentary life so as not to strain that weakened heart. The medical profession was making cardiac cripples out of thousands of people. Now all that is changed. The patient is moved out of the coronary unit of the hospital in a few days to a week. He is then monitored in another hospital room while he is gradually made ambulatory. In a few more weeks, if all goes as expected, an increasingly vigorous exercise program is instituted.

Exercise does several things for the patient:

1. It improves general good health and physical condition.
2. It helps bring body weight into its optimal range, approaching the ideal body weight.
3. It helps restore confidence and hope in the patient, preventing or alleviating the devastating post-coronary depression that normally accompanies heart disease.
4. It keeps the patient from becoming a cardiac cripple.
5. Most important, it helps develop collateral circulation for the heart itself—a system by which small blood vessels coursing through the heart muscle help supply blood and oxygen to the cells of the heart.

If you are a sufferer of heart disease (or any other chronic ailment for that matter), do not take it for granted that the best is behind you and that you are on that great downhill slide to oblivion. Now we know better. Walking is being prescribed more and more often by knowledgeable physicians and other health professionals to bring people back from the brink of death to vigor and robust good health. IF YOU HAVE HAD A HEART ATTACK, USE WALKING TO PREVENT ANOTHER. Your successful rehabilitation can greatly depend on a good, supervised walking program.

Quoting the famed Dr. Kenneth Cooper in relation to what happens when walking is used for rehabilitation of cardiac patients, he says: "Aerobic exercise increases the cells of your

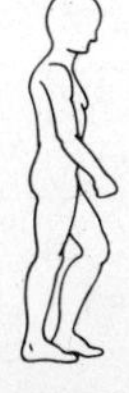

body. New vessels may appear as if from nowhere—perhaps because of the physical stimulus of the vigorous circulation or perhaps by some chemical trigger. We don't know the cause, but the result is that when you get your heart rate up during an aerobic exercise workout, the cells throughout your body get a better cleansing and more life-sustaining oxygen than they did before."

Apparently the phenomenon of collateral circulation, in which new pathways bypass restricted areas of the arteries and provide additional circulation to the heart, is one of the benefits of aerobic exercise. Studies at the UCLA medical school have demonstrated that more than 75 percent of angina pectoris patients improved drastically through a carefully monitored walking program. The angina pains totally disappeared in several of the patients, eliminating completely the need for nitroglycerine medication. Once collateral circulation begins to develop, there is no telling how far you can go.

Attend the Honolulu Marathon, held annually in December, and see as many as 40 or 50 postcardiac patients enter and successfully complete the 26-mile marathon under the direction of their famed cardiologist, Dr. Jack Scaff. When these people with their broken-heart T-shirts finish the race, they receive more applause than the world-class athletes. The reason for their success is the careful monitoring of each individual patient as he progresses from cardiac cripple to full-fledged marathoner. Walking is the key to getting started in any ambitious program such as this to gain the necessary endurance.

If you do have any sort of a heart problem, take this book and show it to your cardiologist. Tell him you want to get into the best physical shape possible. Let him prescribe a safe walking program for you and then let him monitor your progress. Perhaps he will stress-test you on a treadmill periodically to see how your heart strength is improving and to increase your safety.

As you work out, the system of collateral circulation around your major arteries is increasing, making your chances of survival many times greater than those of your sedentary counterparts. Strong, healthy hearts conditioned by exercise can pump much more oxygenated blood with each stroke. During our lifetimes we circulate more than 100 million gallons of blood through our bodies with a little one-pound pump we call our heart. If we are wise, we will all do everything we can to keep it in excellent working order.

Dr. Terrence Cavanaugh, director of the Toronto Rehabilitation Center, has been working with recovering heart attack victims for many years with great success. He has found that faithful exercisers have a much lower incidence of repeat heart attacks. He says that the fascinating aspect of rehabilitating those who have had cardiovascular problems is that putting them into aerobic exercise programs has caused them to become more fit than ever before in their lives. You could even say that their heart problems were the beginning of new and better lives for them—almost a blessing in disguise.

If you have had a coronary bypass operation, your cardiologist will undoubtedly want you too to undertake an aerobic exercise program. Walking should best fill your needs. Let your doctor prescribe your beginning program. If you smoke or depend on any other chemicals harmful to your health, ask him to help you kick the habit. In addition, discuss your eating habits with him. We will wager that he will wish you to conform to our suggestions in Chapter 9, "Your Healthy Diet." For best results, you, your health professional and this book should become a team dedicated to your health and longevity.

## Arthritis

Arthritis is a real crippler and a great disincentive to exercise. There are many forms of arthritis, but most affect us in the same way—they cause us pain and limitation of motion in our joints. When it hurts to move a joint, the natural thing to do is stop moving it; but the problem is, that causes the joint to become more limited in motion and more painful when we are forced to use it. The painful fact is that to avoid joints becoming completely immobile through disuse and atrophy, they must be kept as flexible and mobile as possible with a combination of anti-inflammatory agents and movement.

Some people have such severe cases of arthritis that they must walk in swimming pools in order to keep the weight off their joints, especially if they are overweight. When cases are

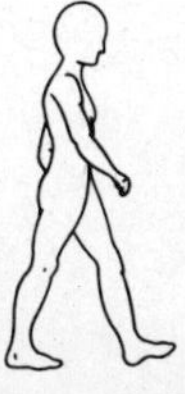

in an extremely severe period, it is important that exercise be very mild. One must not give up, however, because improvement can almost always be made.

Pain and immobility are such individual things for each arthritis sufferer, it is impossible to generalize how much exercise to do. First get the advice of your health professional. The amount and intensity of exercise can be likened to that of the heart patient who is also gradually overcoming a very serious disease. Perhaps the initial exercises must be of a passive type rendered by a therapist. But gradually, even people with acute cases are able to get out and walk.

If a person gives up and doesn't exercise at all, this is extremely counterproductive. The affected joints will atrophy and movement will become more and more limited until there will be none at all. SLOW WALKING IS ONE OF THE EASIEST AND MOST NATURAL MOVEMENTS THROUGHOUT LIFE, AND THIS NATURAL MOVEMENT IS VERY BENEFICIAL IN KEEPING AN ARTHRITIS SUFFERER'S JOINTS RELATIVELY MOBILE.

Some severe cases require surgical joint replacement. Modern technology has made replacement hips, knees and other joints very good, comfortable and effective. We have seen people crippled by arthritic hips return to active sports such as tennis, walking, swimming, cycling and other vigorous activities after hip replacement surgery. Knee replacement surgery is by far superior to what it was just ten years ago. A knee prosthesis can take you out of a wheelchair and put you back on your feet in a matter of days if you are suited for this operation and there is no other alternative to surgical correction. Here is a very remarkable example of successful knee replacement: Chuck Hunter of Longmont, Colorado, an avid walker for many years even though his right knee was plagued with degenerative arthritis, decided to have his knee joint replaced with an artificial one manufactured by the T. Richards Company. Since the operation, he has competed successfully in long-distance walking races, including a 100-miler in 1987, without incident.

## Obesity

Obesity abounds in this largely sedentary society, and is a serious problem, since it contributes to a great number of ailments, including hypertension and heart disease. Excess weight contributes to inactivity, and inactivity is a main cause of weight gain. Stress and anxiety lead often to compulsive eating, which leads to obesity, which leads to physical inactivity, which leads to stress and anxiety. We call this a vicious cycle. We contend that physical activity is the best way of breaking this deadly chain of events. It goes without saying that exercise is as important as diet in reducing weight, and ideally there should be a combination of the two. (See Chapter 9, "Your Healthy Diet.")

Some unfortunate souls have a high appestat setting. The appestat is the regulator in the hypothalamus that determines the size of our appetites. High appestats tend to almost always cause obesity unless counteracted by an appropriate calorie-burning exercise. The grossly obese find it extremely difficult to do any exercise at all, but there have been phenomenal successes by those truly motivated to lose weight. Endurance activities such as walking burn glycogen and fat about equally, while the short-burst, high-intensity exercises burn glycogen almost exclusively. WALKING IS ONE OF THE VERY FEW EXERCISES THAT THE TRULY OBESE CAN TOLERATE AND IS THE ONE MOST OFTEN RECOMMENDED BY WEIGHT-LOSS AUTHORITIES.

Those suffering from overweight must work on endurance and not speed until approaching ideal weight. Physical science has shown that just about the same amount of foot-pounds of energy is required to move an object the same distance, whether it is done at moderate speeds or rapidly. This indicates to us that it is distance and not speed that burns most of our calories. In covering a mile it makes little difference whether you run or walk—in either case it takes around 100 calories of energy. The main difference is that it might take eight or nine minutes to jog the distance and 15 or more minutes to walk it. If you are more than pleasantly plump, it is important to walk at a speed that tests you a little but not so fast that it completely exhausts you. Walk as far as you can and keep the speed within the comfort range. Always keep your ideal pulse rate range in mind as you walk; with experience, you can tell without thinking when you are within the range. Keep working until you can increase your endurance up to the point where you can walk for an hour or more each day. The pounds will melt away gradually and consistently. A 50- to 100-pound-loss in a single year is not uncommon for those who religiously follow a good program of diet and aerobic walking, but be aware that loss must be gradual.

## Respiratory Diseases

Obstructive respiratory disease, and in particular emphysema, ranks second behind heart disease as a destroyer of men and women in their most productive years. Most of these respiratory diseases are caused by smoking and are not completely reversible (see Chapter 10, "Fight Killer Habits.") In fact, once air cells (alveoli) are affected by emphysema, they cannot be regenerated and capillaries are destroyed. Total lung volume is increased, but breathing capacity is diminished. Unfortunately, the progression is insidious and tends to get worse and worse unless its progress is halted.

For someone with a respiratory disease, any exercise is very painful, but complete inactivity can be deadly. As painful as the exercise is, it must be done if there is to be any sort of quality of life at all. Inactivity can only make things worse. It takes a lot of courage to overcome the frightening effects that damaged lungs cause (for example, hands may turn blue or swell up), but THE VICTIM OF RESPIRATORY DISEASE CAN MAKE DEFINITE PROGRESS IN INCREASING THE CIRCULATORY SYSTEM'S CAPACITY AND THE BLOOD VESSELS IN THE LUNGS WITH A WALKING PROGRAM.

The walking program should be supervised by a physician and based on very gradual increase, probably even more gradual and with less potential for improvement than that of heart patients. As improvement occurs, it does so only minimally in actual breathing function—the damage is already done—but there can be significant changes for the better in blood circulation to the lungs. Those dedicated to improving can accomplish a great deal more work and be less dependent on others. Gradual is the key word. Speed is not. Patients may be able to walk for only a minute or so at first before becoming very breathless, but as time goes by they may be able to increase the time to as much as a half-hour.

Everyone has concerns about a healthy heart, and rightly so because of the heart-attack epidemic in our country. In comparison, lung disease gets much less attention, and yet it is the lungs that process our staff of life—oxygen—without which we can survive for only a few minutes. Consider these facts:

1. Oxygen energizes every cell of the body. It is the key to the energy chain that keeps us alive.
2. Most of the oxygen we take in is used to maintain cell and tissue structure—the balance is used for muscle functions that are involved in everyday living activity.
3. A shortage of oxygen affects every organ of the body.
4. The brain has the highest oxygen requirement of all the bodily organs; the heart has the second highest.
5. The liver, kidneys and all other organs require oxygen for their own vital functions.
6. In states of oxygen deficiency the whole body becomes robbed of vital energy.

Most of us have periodic checkups covering most of the bodily functions. Yet, if the lungs are so critical to our health and happiness, why do we take them for granted? We must become more aware of their huge importance to our well-being. The amount of air that can be blown out of a fully inflated lung, called the vital capacity, is a better predictor of longevity than any other test, including blood pressure, electrocardiograms or blood tests. It is our capacity for life. Yet very few of us even know what vital capacity is. Let us recognize the lung as the key health organ that it is; we should equate lungs with life. We must learn the condition of our own lungs in order to protect and strengthen them. Walking for health and fitness is surely one of the best ways to boost vital capacity; it strengthens us to survive the rigors of everyday living in good shape and with less effort by increasing our lung power.

Lung disease sufferers can learn to monitor their own bodies as they improve, and eventually accomplish far more than they thought they could. This is a pleasant discovery for those thus afflicted.

## Asthma

An asthma attack, with its labored breathing symptoms, can be frightening. But with proper management and a good walking program, asthmatics can lead active and productive lives. Often victims of this disease must time medication in relation to exercise to avoid complications, especially if they suffer from exercise-induced asthma. It is possible for practically every asthma sufferer to exercise safely with the emphasis on participation rather than on high-level performance. They should go at their own pace.

Cold air temperatures and high amounts of pollen in the air can be limiting factors on the amount of walking done, since severe wheezing may occur. Some asthma sufferers are limited psychologically because they fear pushing themselves too much and developing bronchospasm. But the average exerciser should not worry unduly, because the good effects of exercise far outweigh the bad. Even world-class athletes such as Bill Koch, the best cross country ski racer in the USA for many years, have successfully coped with exercise-induced asthma while competing at a world-class level of competition. If Bill Koch can do that, there is good reason to expect that MOST AVERAGE ASTHMA SUFFERERS CAN FIND A WALKING PACE AND LEVEL OF EXERCISE THAT WILL HELP IMPROVE THE CONDITION TO A MARKED DEGREE.

Studies have shown that after the age of 20, when we are at our maximum powers, we begin to lose an average of 1 percent of our oxygen processing capacity per year. This results in a similar lessening of cellular activity, and our bodies start a long, slow decline toward suffocation. That is, unless we are astute enough to undertake a program of some form of aerobic exercise for the rest of our lives.

According to exercise physiologists, gains in aerobic capacity compared very favorably to what might have been expected from people much younger. Asthma patients can make similar strides in improvement with proper supervision.

## Diabetes

Diabetes is a chronic disease for which walking must have been invented. The person who can maintain an even balance between diet and activity is a person who can control his diabetes. The main problem is the difficulty of maintaining an even level of activity. It is far easier to maintain an even level of food consumption. In sports, many times you don't know if the activity will be strenuous or easy. Walking is, however, completely predictable. When you walk a measured distance each day, you will burn almost the same number of calories each time out. Therefore, WALKING IS THE DIABETIC'S IDEAL EXERCISE, WITHOUT A DOUBT.

Not only is walking predictable but it helps the circulation, especially in the lower extremities—an area where severe diabetics often get into trouble with ulcerations, infections, pain and neuropathies due to deterioration of blood flow. Diabetics must take special care to get only well-fitting and comfortable shoes to wear, to avoid blisters if possible.

There are more than 10 million Americans who have this disease to some degree. It is characterized by the inability of the pancreas to produce a sufficient amount of insulin, or the the inability of the body to use the insulin produced. Dietary sugars, starches and other foods are converted into the sugar called glucose, which is converted to energy by insulin as it is distributed through the bloodstream to the cells.

With Type II diabetes, the adult-onset type, dramatic improvements can be made through a program of diet and exercise. Type I is more difficult to work with, since it begins with a chronic insufficiency of insulin very early in life that normally must be controlled with measured injections. Being physically fit does not prevent Type I from occurring, but exercise can lessen the amount of injected insulin required. Exercise somehow makes it easier for insulin to move glucose out of the blood and into the cells, and this effect can be cumulative as a person gets into better and better shape.

The wise diabetic should make himself an experiment of

one and keep track of diet, amount of insulin injected, miles walked and how he or she feels every day. By keeping track like this one can design an exercise program based on individual experience—which is an excellent way to do it, as we are all different to some degree. You must become familiar with your own metabolism. The more you know, the more you can be in control of the disease, rather than have it control your life. Exercisers frequently find that they need to alter their schedule of insulin injections to fit their exercise programs so as to maintain stable glucose levels. It may be necessary to carry a snack along on longer walks in case low blood sugar sets in. Due to the tendency toward excess urination, diabetics often need an increased fluid intake to avoid dehydration.

Studies have shown that exercise improves glucose tolerance and raises insulin sensitivity, which makes it possible for some Type II diabetics to discontinue the use of insulin, and for some Type I diabetics to reduce their dosage by as much as half. It is vital that you follow your physician's advice in regard to your walking program. Essentially, there is little that a diabetic cannot do so long as he does it methodically with the proper medical advice, assesses cause and effect before and after exercise and makes suitable adjustments as necessary.

## Osteoporosis

Few of us think of bones as living tissue that is affected by exercise. The fact is that BONES DO RESPOND TO THE CORRECT TYPE OF EXERCISE—ESPECIALLY WALKING. As bones receive the stress of weight-bearing exercise and its accompanying muscular contractions and compressional impacts, they respond by taking on more calcium and phosphorus, causing them to become denser, thicker and stronger. The *Nutritional Reports International* published the following statement: "A physically active lifestyle is necessary to induce this calcification. Bone growth and density increase in proportion to the compressional load a bone is asked to carry." It takes only about six days for bones to begin to demineralize in someone who is bedridden, according to a hospital study. Even the modest strain caused by standing still was found in one experiment to retard the rate at which hospitalized patients lost bone density. Walking is a proven exercise to increase bone density because of the way it compresses the bones.

## Cancer

Exercise is now being recognized as a part of cancer therapy, since it makes us stronger physically as well as mentally, emotionally and psychologically. It also tends to keep a person at normal weight.

Studies show that obese women are at a far greater risk of developing cancer than those of normal weight. Obesity can undermine the integrity of the immune system, so it is very important to stabilize weight. Now studies are showing that those of us who achieve and maintain a good physical condition are not only less likely to develop cancer, but are better able to survive should the dread disease develop. IF YOU SHOULD NEED TO UNDERGO CANCER TREATMENT OF ANY TYPE, A GOOD WALKING PROGRAM WILL ENHANCE ITS BENEFITS IN ALMOST ALL CASES. Although you can't walk away from cancer quite as readily as you can from heart disease, there is strong evidence that it is well worth the effort to try to do so. Ideally, all cancer patients should have a regular schedule of exercise commensurate with their ages and physical capabilities.

Vigorous exercise is somewhat incompatible with cigarette smoking and so can help eliminate this insidious habit. Tobacco is probably the worst known carcinogen there is. Specialists say that around 90 percent of all lung cancers are cigarette related. In an experiment at the Labor Science Institute in Japan, mice restricted from exercise developed cancer at a rate of 60 percent, whereas mice forced to exercise developed the disease at a rate of only 23 percent. The exercise group also ate less and proved more resistant to the carcinogen benzidine.

A notable example of someone who fought back against cancer was a young man named Terry Fox, a Canadian. At age 18 he was diagnosed as having osteogenic sarcoma (bone cancer) in his right leg and was told it had to be amputated to save his life. As traumatic as that was to the otherwise healthy

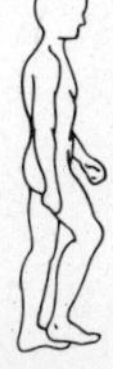

young man, he decided to do everything possible to lick the disease. He read about another above-the-knee amputee named Dick Traum, who had successfully completed the 1976 New York Marathon on one good leg and an artificial one. This motivated him to set up a long-range goal: To walk across Canada to see if someone with this horrible disease could do it, and to get publicity and funds for cancer research. After three years of chemotherapy and endurance training he decided to try. The route started in St. John's, Newfoundland; the destination was Vancouver, B.C. Although he didn't reach Vancouver, he did average 24 miles per day and covered 3,339 miles before he was forced to retire. He was an inspiration to all, and he raised more than $1 million for cancer research. He had carried hope to all cancer victims everywhere and demonstrated that victims of the disease can do amazing things if they really try.

## High Blood Pressure

According to researcher Ralph Paffenbarger, M.D., of Harvard and Stanford universities, hypertensives need not shy away from exercise. In fact, exercise tends to reduce blood pressure and the risk of heart attacks. In an extensive study he found a 35 percent greater risk of hypertension in college alumni with low exercise participation. Another study by epidemiologist Steven Blair demonstrated that EXERCISE HAS A LONG-TERM RESIDUAL EFFECT AS EVIDENCED BY LOWERED INCIDENCE OF HIGH BLOOD PRESSURE LATER IN LIFE. He found that people with low levels of initial fitness were more likely to develop hypertension. It is interesting to note that hypertensive athletes are able to compete successfully at high levels with no apparent adverse effects from their disease. They must use care, however, not to become dehydrated if they are using diuretics to help control the disease.

Although an exercise such as walking can be very beneficial to those with high blood pressure, sufferers should normally avoid isometric or weight lifting exercises, which restrict blood vessels and thus elevate the pressure, possibly to dangerous levels.

## Paralysis

Few paralyzed people will read this book, but developments in this field are so exciting that we felt compelled to include it. RECENTLY, EVEN PARAPLEGICS HAVE BEEN GIVEN THE OPPORTUNITY TO WALK. This is possible with the assistance of computers. Some ingenious experiments by a research team at Wright State University in Dayton, Ohio, have resulted in the ability to hook up electrodes to the non-responsive muscles of the paralyzed victims, and provide the proper stimuli to actually simulate a walking motion in the legs. Jerold Petrofski has been working on such a device since 1968, when he had the idea that it would be possible for mini-computers to simulate central nervous system activity to bypass paralyzing spinal injuries. Petrofski said, "I looked at the problem logically. Your muscles are like a motor in your body, and if you've been paralyzed from the neck down, your brain keeps saying, 'Move,' but the message can't get down to the rest of your body. You have a perfectly functioning system down there. It's just turned off. So the problem is to bring it back up again without blowing it apart."

In 1982 he was able to apply the techniques to humans after years of experimentation on animals. Patience is needed because someone who has sat in a wheelchair for a long time has extremely weak muscles and bones. It takes six months of training to regain bone strength and density, but only two months to regain muscle strength. The bones are extremely fragile at first and subject to fracture, but gradually respond to weight-bearing exercise. One subject was able to settle into a routine of walking 30 minutes steadily three times per week and was remarkably vigorous for someone who was completely paralyzed. This type of experimentation holds great promise for the future of paraplegics and quadriplegics. So you can see there is hope for almost everyone, no matter what their condition. In fact there are no really valid excuses for anyone to remain completely sedentary.

## Headache

Headache is one of the most common complaints of all.

The trouble is that there are so many causes and effects that it is hard to generalize on this subject. It is estimated that perhaps 40 million Americans seek medical help because of the recurring severity of their headaches. Pain is often so intense that work and home life are both severely compromised. Concentration is difficult if not impossible. Scientists have divided headaches into three basic groups: muscle contraction headaches, vascular headaches and a miscellaneous category that includes traction and inflammatory headaches.

The stress in our lives is estimated by experts on the subject to cause around 70 percent of headaches severe enough to warrant medical attention; these are usually of the muscle contraction type. Fortunately, headaches of this type do not last too long and are very often relieved by brisk walking. Exercise has come to be the the most practical release for accumulated tension. Brisk walking dissipates the symptoms of stress, thus preventing headaches, and in some cases, relieves certain types of headaches when it is too late to prevent them. Although muscle contraction headaches are relieved by aspirin and other over-the-counter medications, it is far better for us to get the same results from exercise, which has only good side effects.

Usually the most debilitating type, which comes under the vascular category, is the migraine or cluster headache. In its first phase the constriction of blood vessels in the head and brain reduces blood flow. This is painful and disorienting, with dizziness, weakness, numbness, and visual problems. The second phase is even worse, as blood vessels along the surface of the brain and scalp expand and allow more than usual blood flow. There is often increased pressure over the whole cranium and the pain can be very intense. Although it is next to impossible and unwise to exercise during one of these headaches, studies and numerous case histories have shown that aerobic exercise can reduce the frequency of these painful migraines.

Cluster headaches occur mainly in middle-aged men who smoke or drink alcohol. These attacks are often daily and last around 30 minutes. It is possible to help relieve these headaches by exercising during them, but rapid walking during the pain-free period between attacks can sometimes bring on another headache. According to headache researcher Otto Appenzeller of the University of New Mexico, relief of cluster pains coincides with a surge of natural pain killers called beta endorphins in the body's systems. In addition, the increased circulation caused by exercise has a beneficial effect.

Many headaches in the miscellaneous category caused by any number of things are helped by exercise, but others may not be. Miscellaneous causes may be major or minor medical problems, including brain tumor, meningitis, encephalitis, aneurysm, brain hemorrhage, joint dysfunction of neck or jaw, temporal arteritis (inflammation of artery to scalp) or disease of the eyes, ears, nose or throat. It is essential that you follow your physician's advice for your particular condition as to whether the activity will relieve or worsen your particular type of headache. Remember that acute pain may signal a major medical problem, and medical attention is necessary if the onset of the headaches is recent and is getting progressively worse. Beware if they are sudden, severe and incapacitating, if there is nausea and vomiting, fever and stiff neck, drowsiness, double vision, numbness, weakness, speech or coordination difficulty.

## Stroke

Stroke is another disease in which great strides in knowledge have been made in recent years. Vigorous rehabilitation can do miracles for stroke patients who just a few years ago would have been placed in homes or hospice and left to deteriorate further. Individuals have come back from almost complete paralysis and inability to communicate to become active and productive. A famous example is the actress Patricia Neal. She has recovered fully and is now a spokeswoman for stroke patients. Stroke patients need the courage of their convictions to stick to therapeutic programs until they gain the coordination, strength and confidence to get back in shape with walking programs.

For a stroke patient a walking program may have to start with a single step, but if that single step can be accomplished, then it is possible to take two . . . three . . . and more, and more . . . and more . . . .

## Bad Back

Practically all of us at some period in our lives suffer from back ailments and pain. Something as simple as improper sitting posture can lead to problems. If you slouch over too much there is strain and tension on the back muscles. The back should be held as erect as possible when you are sitting. People who sit for prolonged periods at work or elsewhere experience shortening of some postural muscles, particularly the hamstrings. This should be counteracted by getting up and walking around periodically to stretch out the affected muscles.

A soft bed or one that sags too much in the middle is the back's archenemy. The spinal erector muscles are detrimentally affected during a night's sleep in such a bed. Experts suggest that a piece of plywood should be used under the mattress to eliminate the sag and keep the body in a more natural position.

The chief problem, however, is lack of fitness and muscle tone. While it is true that the back muscles are among the strongest in the entire body, you would never suspect this because of the epidemics of back ailments experienced in the USA. The culprits are the opposing muscles at the front—the abdominals. Most people have notoriously weak abdominal muscles (and many older men have pot bellies). This causes an imbalance and added strain on the back muscles that can cause a pelvic misalignment and a forward tilt at the top. The sacrum (tailbone) also will tilt forward, putting increased pressure on the sacroiliac joint and the ligaments located on the front of the lumbar vertebrae. Weakness in the gluteals and/or hamstring muscles may also cause pelvic tilt. Lordosis can result and a possible "slipped disc" injury that we hear about so often.

How do we tone those muscles to keep them strong enough to avoid muscle imbalances and painful back injuries? Brisk walking is a very good and logical answer.

While you should build up your walking program gradually, strolling too slowly at first will not help much. To gain muscle strength in the hamstrings, gluteals and abdominals, the speed and effort must be such that all these muscles are worked enough to get a training effect. At higher speeds, the nature of the racewalking style works on all three muscle groups. You should feel the hamstrings (not the quadriceps) pushing you forward at the rear of your stride. The gluteal and abdominal muscles are toned as the hips do their characteristic rolling motion. It may be necessary to do supplementary abdominal exercises for strength—it all depends on the effort you put into the speed-walking movements. YOU CAN ALLEVIATE BACK PAIN IF YOU LEARN HOW TO WALK WITH GOOD POSTURE AND WITH ENOUGH INTENSITY.

## Foot Ailments

Although walkers can often get along quite nicely with very ordinary feet, overdoing the exercise may cause some troubling ailments. Following are five of the most common causes of the "Agony of Defeet."

1. OVERPRONATION—The normal foot rolls inward and down when it strikes the surface, to absorb the shock of impact and keep the balance. If the foot rolls in too much the result may be arch pain, inner knee pain or heel spurs. If this occurs an orthotic can often alleviate the problem by returning the foot to its normal motion.

Orthotics—rigid or non-rigid inserts that are placed in the shoe and cast to the shape of your foot—can range in price from $65 to $250 or more, depending on their quality and complexity. Find a well-qualified podiatrist to help you if you find that you cannot solve foot-pain problems by yourself.

2. HEEL SPUR—A projection of bone on the bottom of the heel that may result from improper foot landing or abnormal positioning. Inflammation around this abnormal bone formation often causes pain. The pain, however, is not usually caused by the bone formation itself. In minor cases a simple over-the-counter heel pad may suffice to relieve the pain. Acute cases will probably require a custom-made orthotic by a podiatrist to realign the foot to normal during walking.

3. PLANTAR FASCITIS—The fascia is a thick, inelastic fibrous band that stretches from the metatarsals to the heel. Pain in the arch or heel may be the signal that the fascia is

under too much strain. Since many foot abnormalities can cause strain, you may need to experiment to find relief. Arch supports, heel lifts or stiff replacement inserts may be helpful in this case.

4. ACHILLES' TENDONITIS—This tendon connecting the heel bone to the calf muscles may be too inflexible to stand the strain of a lot of walking It can become inflamed, irritated and extremely painful. Heel lifts are often the solution to this problem.

5. SESAMOIDITIS—If there is a sharp pain in the ball of the foot, this ailment may be indicated. This condition occurs when two tiny bones in the foot below the metatarsals become bruised. Over-the-counter padded inserts can relieve the pressure in all but the most severe cases; otherwise, orthotics are necessary to correct the condition.

It takes time, patience and sometimes money to correct foot problems. But when you consider the benefits of walking for your health, it is well worth working on a solution to the painful ailments that can be so discouraging.

## Should We Exercise When Under the Weather?

Exercises such as walking can definitely make you feel better if the cause of your distress is from some external source causing tension, worry or fatigue. Exercise in these cases can have a very calming and beneficial effect. Beware, however, of over-exercising if the source of feeling bad is from systemic disease. The whole basis of getting stronger and healthier through exercise is that it is done in such an intelligent way that the muscles and tissues tired by exercise have time to recover before the exercise is undertaken again. In this case, muscle tone and strength will gradually increase.

Tissue protein must be replaced to effect the rebuilding and strengthening process. Under the ideal conditions of exercise and rest afterward, a person will synthesize more muscle protein than he lost. If he over-exercises without sufficient rest between bouts, there is a net loss of muscle protein and an ensuing weakening effect. Exercise takes energy, and it is wise not to cut calories so far that the weakening effect happens too often. Authorities suggest as a rule of thumb that average-size men should not eat less than 1,500 calories daily and women not less than 1,200. If calories are too limited, the protein in the diet will automatically be converted to glucose and fat for energy, and it won't be available for biosynthesis.

If you are sick systemically, the tissue-repairing ability of the body is decreased by the fact that the body is fighting the illness. If you have a sore throat, you must decide whether or not it is from yelling at a sporting event, too much time in a smoke-filled room, or a symptom of flu. The first two will not preclude your normal exercise, but the third definitely should—the flu will retard regeneration no matter what the exercise is. Emotional stress can also reduce recuperative processes. Protein eaten during emotional stress is not utilized well, which is demonstrated by the fact that there is a distinct increase in protein waste in the urine. All the factors are cumulative. If you are suffering from some mild systemic disease, emotional problems and poor diet all at the same time, your exercise will do you little good until you become rested enough to recover.

Unfortunately, the older you are the more the problems are magnified and the more careful you have to be not to get overstressed. Recuperative processes are slowed. You may not recover in a day from your exercise, and walking may be better for you—if done briskly only every other day. Sometimes people over 60 or 70 have gone into well-intentioned exercise programs only to suffer a net muscle loss by overextending themselves. Illnesses seem to be magnified in their effects on older people, especially if they have not stayed in shape throughout life. Extra care must be taken to keep tissue repair ahead of the tissue damage. This is not to discourage the older person from walking—since it must be done to stay in shape—but only to warn against doing too much too soon until the body is accustomed to vigorous exercise.

We allow ourselves to succumb prematurely to a wide spectrum of diseases, many of which can be alleviated by the benefits inherent in a brisk walking program. Here we have covered those encountered by the most people. If you have a disability, don't go down in defeat. Where there is life there is hope, and remarkable recoveries happen all the time. Everyone can set realistic goals to achieve. Regardless of how slow progress seems in the beginning, the effort will reap results faster than you realize. Many health professionals are recommending brisk walking to their patients. Brisk walking can more often than not be the best prescription for what ails you, and the side effects are outstanding in a favorable sense.

Start today if you haven't already done so!

# CHAPTER 14

# WALKING AND RETIREMENT

*"The next major advance in the health of the American people will come from the assumption of individual responsibility for one's own health, and a necessary change in lifestyle for a majority of Americans."*

—John Knowles, M.D.,
President, Rockefeller Foundation

---

Retirement may seem to be a long way off for many of you, but as years go by you will realize that life is short—often too short to do all the things that you dream of when you have time. Some think that making wise financial investments when young will be the total answer to happy and carefree retirement. We contend that making an investment in your personal health is far more important. What good are all the riches in the world if you are too unhealthy or infirm to enjoy them? When young you must invest wisely not only in financial matters but also in your own personal health, and maintain this throughout the years until the time comes to quit working for a living. Then you can cash in on your investment of lifetime fitness through brisk walking and continue to be just as active, or even more so, during retirement as when young. You may feel just fine now, and can't imagine decrepitude in old age, but it can be very real unless you think ahead and take action now.

Have you ever noticed how an apparently healthy and spry person deteriorates in a very short time after retirement from his lifelong job? Is the deterioration physical or psychological? Actually it is both. It may begin as psychological, which then leads to the physical decline, which leads to an early demise. It is a sad situation and such a waste. Many people work hard all their lives, looking forward to a carefree, restful retirement. But before they have a chance to enjoy those fruitful post-labor years, a nursing home or the grave interferes with all those dreams and plans. Our advice is: reorganize and reprioritize your life. Above all, keep busy!

## Stay Active with Labors of Love

Those folks who truly enjoy their golden years will tell you: "I'm busier now than I ever was when I worked for my living." Trade your labor for survival in for a labor of love. It's all right to get up an hour or two later than you did when you were part of the work force, but don't spend the rest of the day in your pajamas. Get out and do things—maintain a busy schedule full of things you love and want to do.

We recently met an individual who perfectly illustrates many of the principles we are talking about. Don Cieber is a retired writer from the *Denver Post.* At 64 years of age, he found himself in terrible physical condition as 1986 began. He had been gaining too much weight over a period of several years, and his physician harangued him at each appointment, saying he really should try to lose a lot of weight. He is fairly tall, but at 249 pounds he was, without question, obese. Joint pain from osteoarthritis and high blood pressure were gradually becoming worse as his weight escalated. Even though his friends didn't think he looked all that bad, he knew that his clothes were disguising his flabbiness and that his quality of life had been slipping away. He resolved to correct the conditions with positive actions.

In January 1986 he enrolled in a senior men's fitness class at the North Jeffco Recreation Center in suburban Denver, and also started walking short distances in his residential area—very short distances at first, but gradually increasing to longer circuits as conditioning improved. He started walking up and down hills and gradually increased speed. During this initial training period he modified his diet to reduce substantially the use of salt, sugar, dairy products and red meats—substituting fresh fruit, raw vegetables and fish.

At North Jeffco each Monday he kept track of his progress by noting his weight and pulse rate after his aerobic and stretching exercises. He found that he could consistently drop between one and two pounds per week by staying absolutely consistent with his training program. By August 1986, he had lost precisely 54 pounds (more than the average person can effectively lose in such a short time period) plus eight inches from his waistline. He didn't relish looking like a trim athlete in fat man's clothes, so he bought new ones. His doctor decided that he could discontinue all previously prescribed medications, since all symptoms had completely disappeared. His resting heart rate had decreased to a marvelous 44 beats per minute—a sure sign that his heart had been strengthened to a large degree. His blood pressure had plummeted to 130/70 which is considered normal for anyone of any age. All his joint pains disappeared, and he had far more energy for everyday activities. Seldom will you see such rapid improvement prompted by any exercise and diet regimen, but this story shows what can be done with persistence and dedication.

Don was present when our walking club, The Front Range Walkers, helped on a 5k pledge walk at a shopping mall in November 1986. He joined in and posted a speedy time of 33:31, the second-best time of all, using a rather inefficient hiking style rather than racewalking. If he had known the technique of racewalking, he surely would have walked much faster.

He continues to walk at least four miles per day and prefers to walk outdoors, but uses shopping malls in case of inclement weather. Don says: "I must say that I enjoy a little bit of competition, but fitness walking and the pleasure of being fit are the real reward. I've heard that walking is the fastest growing sport—and I believe it! Each day I see more walkers in my area, and I also believe that there are more walkers—more women than men—than runners in my area. Anyone can walk, and it is a natural activity. All you need to get started is a determination to get going and the discipline to stick with it. Enrolling in a fitness class such as the one I attend gives me an incentive and a schedule to meet. The results are well worth the effort."

Another inspirational example of someone who refuses to submit to old age is Hulda Crooks. At 91, nicknamed "Grandma Whitney," this little dynamo of a woman from Loma

Linda, California, is still taking long hikes and climbing 13,000- and 14,000-foot mountain peaks. She has climbed the highest peak in California (14,494 feet) 22 times since 1962. This climb is 10.5 miles of constant upward trail. She is one of the most legendary figures in California for her hiking exploits and indomitable spirit at an advanced age. But she does not think of herself as old. Fitness and age are completely compatible in her opinion. She says: "There is nothing special about me. I just work at health instead of whiling away my time sitting in a rocking chair."

She was a mere 66 years old when she decided to improve her life through exercise, and that was the year of her first ascent of Mt. Whitney in 1962. In 1970 she had a particularly rough time making it to the summit, so she decided to step up her training regimen, which had not been very strenuous up to that time. She added more miles and a great deal of stair climbing to her training. By means of increased training, her endurance, muscle power and circulation improved to a marked degree. She no longer experienced cold feet in bed at night, and her long mountain hikes became much easier. In 1987 (at 91) she went to Japan at the invitation of a group of Japanese hikers to scale Mt. Fuji. Although slowing down a little and resting more between her hikes, Hulda at last report was planning to keep on truckin', and will not give up even if she can go only partway up the mountain as age inevitably takes its toll.

## Set Your Priorities

Reprioritize your life, and at the the very top of the list place your health. When it goes you are in deep trouble. Everything else in life will go with it if it is lost. Do you think that billionaire Howard Hughes enjoyed the last years of his life cooped up as a junkie recluse, a paranoid shell of his former self, sitting there with all his wealth in his hotel in total seclusion, and yet dying of malnutrition and drug use? His billion dollars meant nothing except to those trying to get a part of it, and he existed in misery for several years before painfully passing on.

Get out and walk every day faithfully and you will remain middle-aged physically and psychologically for the rest of your life. Heed our previous chapters and do the things we advocate. You are now in charge. You are captain of your own ship, so stay at the helm and guide yourself in a healthy course through the retirement years. Schedule two hours a day to get into and stay in shape. This investment in time is even better than a financial investment, because the odds and rewards are a sure thing. Get out and take time to appreciate nature: look at the flowers, the birds and clouds. You may want to get to know the neighbors. Retirement is a time for sociability and enjoyment—if you stay in shape physically and mentally.

You may wish to decrease the intensity of your walking program as time goes by, but conversely, now that you don't need to go to the office every day, you may find that you have the opportunity to get into the best shape of your life. You can concentrate on endurance, which is the best thing you can do. You may develop the endurance to last to a healthy 100 years of age. Speed is not nearly as important as endurance. As a matter of fact, speed does no good anyway unless there is a base of endurance behind it.

Dr. Seiden started walking seriously after trying to push himself as fast as possible through 5ks and 10ks. However, after a while, he gradually gravitated to ultra-distance walks, which suit him better—and he is quite good at those. Bob Carlson got interested in walking in 1971 when Bruce MacDonald brought his racewalking training team to Boulder, Colorado, prior to the Munich Olympic trials. Bruce gave lessons in racewalking to the fitness enthusiasts there, and Bob got excited about the idea of a new sport. He has combined it with long-distance running ever since, although he enjoys the walking a great deal more. (There is more about this fascinating sport in Chapter 8, "Racewalking" and in "Useful Information for Walkers.")

Perhaps you would like to know how our workouts go. Dr. Seiden, in his early 50s, walks about an hour or so four days a week, at a pace that keeps the pulse rate at about 130 to 140. This for him gives a mile pace of 13 to 14 minutes per mile. This normally means a little under five miles plus a cool-down walk at the end. On those four days he gets a good aerobic workout, burning off about 500 calories in each session. On the remaining three days he goes slower for about six miles, at about 15 minutes per mile. At that rate the pulse rate is about

120 beats per minute. These walks burn about 600 calories. Sometimes he slows even further and walks for two hours at about a 16-minute mile. He calls them his mental or nature walks, during which he enjoys the landscape and his surroundings. He has completed several ultra-distance walks of 50 miles and feels that his superb endurance is the key to his enjoyment of "the good life."

On the other hand, Bob Carlson, born in 1924, has been a high-level exerciser since 1967 (he has run 28 marathons) and has no rigid pattern of exercising at all; he goes by the feel of what his body seems to call for to keep in condition. This relaxed attitude makes things all the more pleasant, especially since he can still walk a 20k (12.4 miles) at about a 10-minute-per-mile pace without worrying about any rigid schedule. He does a tough workout when a good race turns up, which seems to be almost weekly in the Colorado hotbed of racing. Years of working on efficient, relaxed racewalking technique are the key in Bob's case. Unless you have been athletic for many years, we recommend that you follow a schedule similar to Dr. Seiden's rather than to Bob's.

All individuals should gauge their speed by their own ideal pulse rates. If you are not already in acceptable shape and where you want to be aerobic-wise, you shouldn't delay in getting started. Do not expect to abuse your body for many years and then hope that money, doctors and pills will bail you out of all your health problems. Nearly everyone is perfectly capable of improving personal fitness and health, but you must be willing to apply yourself. And when you get right down to it, it is basically very simple: a walking program, an intelligent diet and a refusal to poison yourself with smoke and lethal chemicals. We all have remarkable recuperative potential, but if you have been doing less than desirable things to your body in the past 20 or 30 years, you can't expect nature to correct all these wrongs without some effort on your part.

## Endurance Is the Key

The young can be marvelous at sports that require quick reflexes, strength and speed. Oldsters, on the other hand, can be just as marvelous at activities that require endurance and perseverance. Astute mature people across the country are now walking miles and miles, day after day, enjoying the health benefits of the exercise. Larry O'Neil of Montana competed successfully in several 100-mile national walking championships after he was 60 years old and did them in less than 24 hours. Most of the rest of us can stay in very good shape if we spread that distance over a month's time rather than a day's.

The most common difference between an elderly person who can barely shuffle along and one who still walks like a young person is that the latter has remained active throughout life and has retained hip flexibility. There are few disease processes that will immobilize us faster than immobility itself. Disuse causes your hips, muscles, bones, coordination, confidence, timing, balance, endurance and attitude to deteriorate. Hence the "old age shuffle." That is why we consider sedentariness as the disease of disuse. Bringing vigorous activity back into your daily routine will not only halt but may actually reverse most of these problems.

Attend any Senior Games, a competitive series of activities for people over 55, held throughout the nation, and you will see people who have decided the rocking chair in front of the TV set is not the normal way to spend the declining years. More and more people in their 60s to 80s are participating instead of sitting. They are the role models for their peers. They show us we can make the retirement years almost anything we want to make of them. We implore you not to be a constant spectator. You must be a participant in life to be healthy and happy. You can, indeed, be middle-aged both mentally and physically for the rest of your life if you walk enough.

Here is a shocking fact: Almost one in 10 Americans over the age of 65 is in a nursing home, helpless to some degree and needing others to minister to his basic needs. But in Europe the ratio is more like one in 160. Part of that is due to the closer family ties among Europeans, but a bigger part is the attention given to a more active lifestyle. They, as a general rule, do much more walking and physical recreation than those in our affluent society.

We must continually set new goals for ourselves. Without new goals we will lose our sense of worth and purpose. We will sink into depression, sit around feeling moody and useless. We will wake up in the morning with nothing to look forward to except rocking before the TV set, snacking, drinking, smoking and feeling sorry for ourselves, bitter at the world that has left us behind, out of sight, out of mind. Well, that is not the way it is. The world has to go on. Those of you who haven't been forgotten and left behind are those who have stepped out on your own and made the world keep pace with you. Instead of letting yourself fall into depression and disrepair, you have made the effort to keep yourself physically active and mentally alert. Nothing was given you; you made your own good fortune. Good health is rarely a matter of luck—fitness never is.

How do you think that some of the famous oldsters of history made their mark? They didn't create their marvelous achievements by sitting around. It is sad that most present-day people think their lives are just about over when they retire. But consider these examples: Goethe finished writing *Faust* at 82 years of age; Verdi composed his *Requiem Mass* at 87; Leopold Stokowski was conducting symphony orchestras at 89; Michelangelo and Titian were painting masterpieces at 90; P. G. Wodehouse published a novel at 90; Eubie Blake was still playing ragtime on the piano in his late 90s; and Grandma Moses was still painting pictures at 100 years of age.

Bob Carlson saw Lowell Thomas skiing in the high altitude of Colorado when he was 85. Jack Rabbit Johansen (1875-1987) did a great amount of cross country skiing for several years after turning 100, and died finally at 112. Larry Lewis (1867–1973) of San Francisco was still running and walking six miles a day at 105. These were all active people who didn't let a little thing like chronological age bother them. They enjoyed life to the fullest and did not give up on it.

We must all try to stay fit physiologically and psychologically for the rest of our lives until our weakest links fail and cause our demises. It behooves the wise person to identify his weakest links, if possible, and figure out ways to strengthen them. Brisk walking is a good strengthener for most of the systems of the body.

## Practical Uses of Your Fitness

Suppose you wish to use some of your hard-earned retirement money and travel abroad. Would you rather carry a bag full of medicines and pills as your insurance against illness—or a couple pairs of well-broken-in walking shoes as preventive medicine? Think of how enjoyable it would be to be able to walk around all day long and experience at close range the very essence of cultures that you have never experienced before. When you experience foreign countries through a bus window, it is hardly better than looking at a bunch of pictures. When you are mingling with everyone on the street, you are experiencing all the excitement, sights, sounds, smells and the very essence of the place. You see nearly everything that there is to see when moving at two or three miles per hour.

How can you see all the things you came to see if you are too decrepit to walk for any distance? People go to the Louvre in Paris, spend all day walking through it and find that they have gone only about halfway. What chance does the non-walker have to experience that place unless someone pushes him around in a wheelchair? Experienced walkers have a good deal of flexibility both in their joints and in what they can do. They are mobile—not restricted to only the places wheels can go. They can hike up to one of the huts or inns on the Matterhorn if they choose to do so. They can see Venice, where there are no cars or buses at all, up close. The world is theirs.

Dr. Seiden's mother, who is in her 80s, flew to China with a tour group of mixed ages. While people 20 years younger than she sat on the tour bus and waited, she and a few active others walked for more than an hour along the crest of the Great Wall. She went right along with the rest of the group and didn't slow them down a bit. She didn't become spry by sitting in a rocking chair watching TV. When she was 60 she became a widow, and instead of bemoaning her fate and sitting around feeling sorry for herself, she started taking college courses. She signed up for concert series and plays, became a volunteer driver for the blind and still keeps house for herself. A veritable dynamo, she entertains her friends often and thoroughly enjoys all her children, grandchildren and great-grand-children. The only sadness in her life is having to watch so many of her inactive friends give themselves over to illness and untimely demise. Bob's mother, in her mid-90s, keeps active in the Catholic church by attending daily mass and a social breakfast afterward with her circle of friends. She also does her own housekeeping and uses an exercycle for her main form of exercise.

The nay sayers will point to the above examples and state, "They are the lucky ones who have good genetic ancestry." Don't listen to that old cop-out! Most of the disabilities suffered by people over 70 years of age are from acquired diseases not necessarily related to chronological age. The first step in managing many of these health problems of the aged is to recognize that they are merely illnesses to be cured and not a harbinger of worse diseases to come. Illness is a good motivational reason to get well and bounce back with exercise and good health practices, not a reason to give up and let the illness get the best of you.

Some authorities on gerontology have put forth the notion that if the true aging processes and deterioration by unrecognized disease were not accompanied by disuse, our viable life spans could be lengthened considerably. Many of the disabilities experienced by people over 70 years of age are from acquired defects not necessarily related to chronological age. You may think that only those with long-lived ancestors can be strong, vigorous and healthy in old age. This is not necessarily true, however. The first step in managing many health problems is to recognize that they are illnesses to be cured and not just the effects of time.

According to gerontologist Dr. Theodore Klumpp, heredity is not the greatest indicator of personal health, even though it repeats internal physical or chemical patterns of action or reaction. Studies conducted on people who were vigorous and healthy in later life found that genetic similarities were not among the major common characteristics. What this all means is that the majority of us, regardless of our ancestors, have a fighting chance to counteract the ravages that commonly attack people in their retirement years.

## Walking and Patriotism

Have you ever thought that staying in shape and in good health might be a patriotic gesture? Think about it. Health care costs are now costing us around 12 percent of our gross national product and are rising—approaching $400 billion per year. As you might surmise, a disproportionate amount of this huge expenditure is relegated to Medicare, nursing homes, prolonged hospital stays and extraordinary measures to keep terminally ailing elderly bodies alive. Bob Carlson's own chain-smoking uncle was kept alive artificially with a respirator when his lungs ceased to function—at a cost of $38,000 for two weeks of suffering before they let him go. This sort of artificial living must be happening thousands of times per year at great monetary and human-misery costs. His older brother (by 15 years), Ernie Walter, a non-smoker, is approaching 100 years of age and remains an active walker and the "life" of his retirement home in Seattle, Washington. This reinforces the theory that habits and not genetics are the most important predictor for a vigorous old age.

Those over 65 constitute around 10 percent of our population, but more than 30 percent of all funds spent on health care are spent on this group. If present trends continue, our country could be threatened with an inability to keep up with the huge costs in the next century. Every retired person who keeps himself in good shape and healthy—who thus avoids adding to the staggering cost of health care—is doing one of the most patriotic things imaginable: helping to keep costs within reason and the country's financial health viable.

There is an amazing statement made by one of the country's leading cardiologists in the December 1984 issue of *Atlantic* magazine, to the effect that 90 percent of those $25,000 coronary bypass operations done so routinely these days do not extend a patient's life at all. When you consider just how many thousands and thousands of these operations are done each year, you realize that this is an astounding statistic that would be amazing if only HALF true. Although Medicare pays for some of our ills in the retirement years (at great cost to our society), it does not pay for everything, by a long shot, if our health is deteriorating. We can certainly find better things to do with our hard-earned nest eggs than pay medical costs caused by lack of preventive measures taken to avoid disease and disabilities. The tragedy of all this is not in pure cost alone but in how many of the funds are misdirected. Health care for the aged does not prevent the spread of contagious diseases and does not restore functional capacity or well-being in most cases. The money for the most part goes to nursing homes or hospices, pain-reducing drugs, postponing death and prolonging agony.

"Meals on Wheels," which is supposed to be such a boon for the elderly, is actually a detriment in many cases. This type of service and many technological devices used to "make life easier" are sometimes part of the problem. They can be taking away an endeavor that helps keep a person active. Something must be done to change our health care policies for the elderly to focus on nutrition and physical activity in lieu of inactivity and drugs.

## Don't Retire from Life

We must stay busy and active after our jobs. Association with others is most important, as is mutual support. Organizations such as the American Association of Retired Persons (AARP), which you can and should join after the age of 50, are doing much to help make retirement better for us through education, lobbying for legislation and providing a voice for our growing minority.

We all need hobbies, only one of which should be walking. Get involved in social causes, volunteer work or even start a new career for yourself. The authors of this book have done just that. Stay busy and active. Find people with like interests.

Join a walking club or start one if there is none. In "Useful Information for Walkers," we give you advice on starting a club. Walking partners will keep you going and add delight to the exercise. Time literally flies when you are walking with someone else. And you will find that your communications improve. If you walk for an hour it will turn into an hour-long conversation as you enjoy the great outdoors.

Pets need exercise too. You would be hard pressed to find a more eager and loyal walking partner than your faithful dog.

Do you know that statistics show that pet owners live longer than non-pet owners?

We hope that this chapter has convinced you that the retirement years can truly be "golden." When you consider the fact that such a simple thing as brisk walking can cure so many of the ills of mankind with an investment of only 45 minutes or an hour each day, it is amazing that not everyone is taking advantage of this high-return, low-cost investment in personal health. The word is now being spread, however, and with each passing year we are confident that the streets and walkways will become more and more loaded with young and elderly pedestrians walking away from old age. The more you enjoy life, the more life will enjoy you.

## CHAPTER 15

# ON FINDING THE IDEAL HEALTH PROFESSIONAL

*"A person should walk prior to the meal until his body begins to be warmed. Anyone who lives a sedentary life and does not exercise, even if he eats good foods and takes care of himself to proper medical principles—all his days will be painful ones and his strength shall wane."*

—Maimonides

---

If you have been sedentary, have had severe medical problems or have been a smoker for the past several years, you should seek professional help before you enter into a vigorous walking program. At least let that professional know that you are planning to turn your life around physically, and ask whether he wishes to advise you. Actually take this book with you so that your medical advisor will be aware of the program outlined herein. Then you can be advised as to whether there are any parts of the program you should be wary of. This is especially true if you have recently been ill, had surgery or been under a physician's care for any acute or chronic condition. (If you have special chronic health problems, make sure you read the chapters "Killer Habits" and "Disabilities" before you shop for your health care team.)

Let us emphasize the fact that you must get the input from your medical advisor and make this a cooperative project. Your future health is a joint responsibility for both of you, but the emphasis is on YOU. The professionals can give you all the advice in the world, but only you can do the work that is necessary to regain and maintain your health, happiness and productivity.

It is our opinion that "sedentarianism" should be classified as a disease that is in dire need of corrective measures. There are a few rare situations in which avoidance of exercise might be indicated, or the commencement of exercise might need to be closely monitored. But if your advisor insists that you avoid exercise, make him explain to you why. If you are not satisfied with the explanation, don't hesitate to get a second opinion. In the rare case that exercise is proven to be not prudent, follow the advice for now but keep checking as time goes by to see when it can become a part of your life. There are many chronic conditions that respond very well to walking programs. (See Chapter 13, "Overcoming Disabilities" and Chapter 10, "Fight Killer Habits.")

If you are over 35 years of age and not already in condition, are overweight and/or are living a sedentary life, ask your advisor if a cardiac stress test is indicated. This is a test carried out on a treadmill which very precisely increases the physical stress you are undergoing while you walk at increasing speed and steepness. As you walk the treadmill, your heart and respiration will be monitored by an electrocardiograph machine and a device to measure your breathing volume and oxygen consumption. A cardiac stress test on a treadmill gives your physician an objective method in which to set your baseline limit safely. The doctor can then advise you how rapidly you should progress and can also measure your progress as your condition improves. You can even have a very beneficial program under the supervision of a cardiologist or heart surgeon if you have had a heart attack and bypass operation. Show this book and discuss your walking program step by step. It will be extremely unlikely that they will discourage you from undertaking this program. More and more physicians and other health professionals are recognizing walking to be the safest and best post-cardiac type of exercise.

The world-renowned Swedish exercise physiologist, Per-Olof Astrand, has said that it is those who have chosen to lead a sedentary life who need extensive testing to see if they can survive their debilitating lifestyles. They are the ones who are in danger if some sudden emergency comes up. They are in far worse straits under stressful circumstances than someone who is in shape. It is you sedentary folk who most need the advice included in this chapter.

## Choose Your Advisor with Care

If you are like some of us, you may not have been to a doctor or other health advisor in years. You may not even have a regular doctor. Take time and care in finding the best advisor possible for YOU. It is a sad fact that most people spend less time selecting a physician than they do shopping for shoes or a home appliance. Don't you think that your health and happiness should take precedence in this case? It is important that you find Dr. Right for your own particular needs. There are plenty of good doctors and other health professionals to choose from.

How do you find Dr. Right? We will tell you how in this chapter. The problem is finding one who is best suited to help you and advise you in your quest for health. Even though, as we say elsewhere in this book, you are largely responsible for your own well-being, most of us still need a competent professional's help in acute emergencies and for preventive ideas and advice.

Though your neighbor may have the ideal physician for his situation, that particular one may be all wrong for you. We are all different, with different needs; we each make different demands on our doctors. To find the perfect health care professional for you might—should—require several interviews. Yes, we said interviews. You wouldn't hesitate interviewing several people to clean and care for your home. If you are in business, do you immediately hire the first job applicant that comes in? Don't you think it is more important to interview someone who will care for your health? You must live in that body for the rest of your days. If it gets destroyed or badly damaged, where will you live? Many doctors expect people to shop around for their health care. It is the smart thing to do.

For example, if you are past middle age, you may find that a physician or other advisor close to your own age is easier for you to relate to. On the other hand, another one recently trained in gerontology (the science of aging), with all the recent developments at hand, may be more what you need. Only you can make a decision like this. Definitely, you don't want to pick a health care provider who feels that anyone over 50 is over the hill and should take it easy. You want one who tells you that when you go over the top of the hill you can pick up speed going down the other side.

AARP (American Association of Retired Persons) and the Prudential Life Insurance Company have put out a helpful checklist titled: "Give Your Doctor a Routine Examination." In it they state: "It's important to get to know your doctor well. After all, he will be making some of the most important decisions in your life. He should be sensitive to your needs. You should feel comfortable with him." They go on to say: "Speak frankly to your doctor about what concerns you, not just what ails you. Don't be afraid to ask questions." It is amazing to us how many people are hesitant to speak candidly to their physicians. IF YOU CAN'T TALK TO YOUR PHYSICIAN COMFORTABLY YOU PROBABLY HAVE THE WRONG ONE. You also probably have the wrong one if you constantly feel that your concerns aren't serious enough to bother him, or that you are an imposition. This is also true with any other type of health professional you might select.

Your health professional's personality can have quite an effect, even if it is only a placebo effect, on the outcome of your condition. If you believe in him and his advice, his treatment is very likely to work. But psychological reasons are not, of course, the only reason to consult someone compatible. You are more apt to follow his orders when you feel that time and effort have gone into the diagnosis—it makes it much easier to comply with distasteful treatment or advice.

To begin your search for Dr. Right, ask around. Talk to friends about their doctors. Don't ask just for a name and phone number. Ask them what they like about their providers and also what they dislike. If he smokes during the interview, it indicates that he has little regard for his own health and possibly less than he should for yours. Does he have excellent rapport with his patients? It is not necessarily true that a doctor that someone else doesn't like will not be good for you.

## Conducting the Search

Many communities have physician referral services where you can be computer matched to physicians with qualities you are looking for. These services are free and also sometimes very helpful. Available at public libraries are the *American Medical Directory* and the *Directory of Medical Specialists*, covering the credentials of all practicing physicians and the postgraduate education that they have received in their specialty. Your local chiropractic association can give you a list of qualified local practitioners. For certain problems, chiropractors may be of more help than physicians, especially in the fields of prevention and musculo-skeletal ailments. These sources may be very helpful in case you have moved to a new locale and you must seek new health professionals. Your present doctor can also be of help in this case.

Unfortunately, none of these sources can tell you about the professional's personality or demeanor, which can be just as important as technical knowledge or advanced specialty degrees. Some services are just marketing devices of hospitals to build up the practices of their own staffs. Others are paid by physicians to build their practices. That does not mean that you can't find Dr. Right through such a service, but be aware of these facts and judge accordingly. All referrals should be the starting point from which you make your shopping list.

There is much advice to be gained from other health professionals who don't happen to have an M.D. (Medical Doctor) or D.O. (Doctor of Osteopathy) after their name but are holistically and ethically motivated. This would include some nutritionists, dieticians, nurses, chiropractors, exercise physiologists, psychologists, podiatrists, and various types of therapists. If you are considering using non-physicians for treatment or advice, we suggest that you use essentially the same process that we have already outlined in this chapter for doctor selection. But be aware that there are charlatans out there in any discipline, ready to take your money for dubious or even harmful treatments and advice. One of the main points about selecting a physician, if you choose to go that route, is his willingness to work with other types of health professionals. Be wary of one who is opposed to consulting or allowing you to consult with other qualified health care providers. No person is all-knowing in this increasingly technical world; new knowledge is being added constantly in all health-related fields at an astonishing rate. No one person can possibly keep up with it all.

## Everyone Should Establish a Physician-Patient Relationship

If you really take care of yourself and feel nearly indestructible, you may not give much thought to the quality of health care available since you rarely have to seek medical help. But when things go awry, as can happen to anyone through accident or illness, your lack of foresight may come back to haunt you.

Of course, if you already have an advisor with whom you have an excellent trusting relationship, don't change. If you do contemplate change, make an appointment to see the one that looks best on paper or who has the best recommendations. Is his office atmosphere warm and friendly? Is *he* warm and friendly? Does he remind you of a pill pusher, or of someone interested in getting at the root of a problem and preventing its occurrence in the future? Ask him if he is willing to talk to you on the phone when he isn't busy. If he makes a good impression at first glance, that is good. Does he treat you with respect? Respect must be mutual in this case. If you are skeptical it is a bad sign, and you should try another appointment elsewhere.

You must not be passive as far as medical care is concerned. Doctors are not gods but humans just like us, and when they don't know something they must admit it. Be assertive and suggest that you and he must work together—you taking the major role in protecting your own health, with him in the background for help in emergencies or problems you can't handle by yourself. He must be open and honest with you and be willing to tell you exactly the pros and cons of every procedure. He must be aware of your concerns in this regard at the outset.

Sadly, preventive ideas and advice have not been the strong suit of physicians until recently, but that is slowly beginning to change as priorities are being reassessed. Prevention is the only real way to combat the oppressive and spiraling health care costs that have the potential of bankrupting us in the future. Prevention is what will keep us functional for long, active and happy futures. You should make sure that the health professional you select has this philosophy. It is far better to keep us tuned up and walking than to wait until we're broken down and then try to fix our neglected bodies.

When you finally find a health care advisor to whom you can talk comfortably, who takes time to make you feel at ease, who makes you feel your problems and concerns are important, who has the same goals as you to keep you fit and running (oops—walking) for years to come, then you've found your Dr. Right. Work with this person. Your health and fitness need to be a team effort and the greatest responsibility of that team effort is yours.

**CHAPTER 16**

# THE PSYCHOLOGY OF WALKING

*"Methinks that the moment my legs begin to move, my thoughts begin to flow."*

—Henry David Thoreau

---

You may ask: "What does psychology have to do with walking?" As a matter of fact, it can have a great deal to do with it. If you use the exercise wisely as a means of achieving fitness and relaxation, many psychological as well as physiological benefits will become your reward for the effort. On the other hand, if you walk only out of necessity, to get from your chair to your wheels to drive to where there is another chair waiting for you, then there are likely to be numerous negative psychological problems.

We repeat, we have become a "wheel/chair society" because of the widespread prevalence of this type of sedentariness. Success in an exercise program breeds success, and failure breeds failure to a large extent. In one case the spiral to the top brings exhilaration, good health and high self-esteem; the other becomes a vicious spiral down to the depths of sedentariness, low body strength, chronic fatigue and low self-esteem. If your body is in good physical shape, your superior health can be a sensuous experience and a true confidence builder. A sedentary existence, on the other hand, may be very discouraging because of low energy levels and general malaise and apathy toward the joy of living.

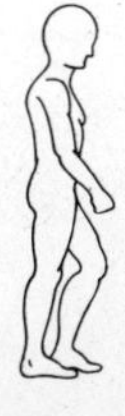

It has been more than amply demonstrated that a vast number of diseases—among people of all ages—are psychosomatic. They originate and feed on themselves in the minds of their victims. People think themselves into either sickness or wellness with the most powerful tool that we all have—our minds. Our psychological tendencies can help or hinder us, depending upon how much we possess them or they possess us. The biggest anxiety producers are our own minds.

Psychological stress can best be defined as the response to a situation created by your view or perception of a circumstance, rather than by the circumstance itself. The great French philosopher Molière once said, "The mind has great influences over the body and maladies often have their origin there." Some thrive on psychological stress while others lose their health from it. It doesn't make any difference whether the stress is real or imagined; it must be reckoned with if the harmful effects are to be neutralized.

There are numerous causes of psychological stress in our lives:

- emotion (anxiety, depression, boredom);
- society (alienation, isolation, overcrowding);
- diet (too much food, too little, wrong type);
- rest (inadequate sleep, overwork);
- health (injury, illness, infection);
- environment (heat and cold, air, water, pollution).

People who are suffering from the lows common to sedentariness should, if they are wise, get into an exercise such as brisk walking to feel better, to improve the appearance of their body, to look younger, to socialize and to improve health. But there are some pitfalls on the way that you should recognize. Lack of time is the most often used excuse for not exercising; but several studies show that the real problem is not using wisely the time already available. Another problem is our modern one of physical laziness caused by overdependence on contrivances to do our work. Participants need to set up for themselves a system of incentives and rewards until the intrinsic benefits of the exercise program become obvious to them. The intrinsic benefits most likely to occur are increase in cardiovascular and general fitness; elevated mood, better relaxation, more energy; weight control; the clearing of one's head; the challenge to improve; relief from overstimulation, overcrowding and the demands of others; and of course, the great physical feeling of walking in an efficient manner.

A good sensible walking program can expand your ability to cope with life and its myriad problems. Fitness can make you less neurotic, more imaginative and more independent. Having a fit body is not a guarantee in itself of emotional well-being. If, however, you are going through the effort to put your body in good shape—to stay trim and energetic—you are going to feel better about yourself than someone who has gone to pot. You will have that extra confidence that enables you to stop worrying about yourself too much. Until you achieve true fitness, don't compete against anyone or anything except your own destructive emotions.

## Mind/Body Relationship Is Not New

As we have mentioned before, the ancient Greeks of around 2,500 years ago realized the close relationship between a sound body and a sound mind, and capitalized on it to produce an advanced civilization and great thinkers and philosophers such as Aristotle, Homer, Plato, Socrates and Hippocrates, the father of modern medicine. Although general awareness of this mind/body relationship apparently was lacking, many of the greatest thinkers throughout history used long walks as a means to collect thoughts in a relaxed, creative manner while their brains were being oxygenated. Examples include Shakespeare, Leonardo da Vinci, Sir Walter Scott (even though somewhat lame), Thomas Jefferson, Jonathan Swift, Henry David Thoreau, Walt Whitman, John Audubon, Thomas Edison, Lewis Mumford. During his term of office, former President Harry Truman used to lead reporters on a merry chase on his regular rapid walks, which he used for relaxation and to relieve his worries about his responsibilities and world affairs. This, of course, was well in advance of the fitness boom, and the ever-present reporters were hard pressed to keep pace with him and were usually too breathless to ask him any questions.

Scientists have determined that the amount of oxygen pumped to our brains over the years has a substantial effect on mental capacity. Researchers from San Diego State University tested the cognitive reaction times of 64 men and women between ages 23 and 59, half of whom were sedentary types and half of whom were habitual aerobic exercisers. They measured how fast each testee could react to an electric stimulus by releasing their index finger from a switch. Cognitive reaction times are known to be excellent indicators of how effectively and efficiently the processes of the central nervous system are working, and they are commonly used to measure degrees of senility for this reason. The sedentary group showed reaction times consistent with their ages. The exercisers, on the other hand, all tested out like youngsters. The researchers then concluded that aerobic exercise seems to strengthen nerve tissue just as it does muscles. The increased enzyme activity and excellent blood flow caused by aerobic exercise appear to safeguard the overall health of the central nervous system and the brain.

A good walk is like a mini-vacation from your troubles. The late Supreme Court Justice William O. Douglas, one of the most avid walking enthusiasts of his time, said that when he had an extremely perplexing legal problem to solve, the most beneficial thing he could possibly do was go out for one of his characteristic long walks. During the walk or soon afterward, a solution or correct answer usually occurred to him almost automatically.

Anxiety is related to tension—though it's like the chicken and the egg as to which comes first. Both can lead to a detrimental spiral of escalating tension and anxiety. If the tension and anxiety are attacked with a regular walking program, the mental state of the walker will improve dramatically. Such a person will perceive that he is taking charge of his life and is actively improving his health, appearance and self-image. There is a feeling of real accomplishment—that depression is being defeated. When enough effort is put into walking to bring it into the aerobic exercise category, the walker will notice significant body sensations that distract him or her. The focus is likely to be on the feelings of movement and mild fatigue, and thus the annoying physical and mental symptoms of depression are left behind.

## Walking Is a Positive Addiction

In time, the exercise of brisk walking, as opposed to all the harmful negative addictions that are so prevalent in our society, can become a positive addiction. Dr. William Glasser has written an entire book on the subject called *Positive Addiction*; it is very worthwhile and enlightening reading. Experience has shown that when depressed people are placed on regular exercise regimens, they experience mood elevation. They feel more relaxed after exercise than before. Some even say that they have experienced an altered state of consciousness, and an opening up of the unconscious—something akin to a dreamlike state.

Dr. Herbert deVries, retired chief physiologist and gerontologist at the University of Southern California, has conducted controlled experiments which demonstrated that a brisk 30-minute walk has roughly the same tranquilizing effect as a standard dose of Valium. Which of these do you suppose has the most desirable side effects? He found not only that a single dose of a tranquilizer had no effect but also that a single bout of exercise had the desired effect. Patients had to take the tranquilizer several times to get relief. But that's not all—in elderly testees, tranquilizers were shown to reduce their reaction time, which was already slowed by the natural effects of aging. This, of course, increases the danger of injury to elderly drivers and the elderly in general who are still functioning in the general mainstream.

The increased blood circulation to the brain and the release of the body's own tranquilizing chemicals (called beta-endorphins) can bring on a feeling of euphoria—an exercise "high." For some, though, it may take 40 minutes or so of continuous rhythmic exercise to achieve this state, and on some days it may not occur at all. When it does occur, you feel as though you can walk forever.

Energy levels will increase through training, and there will be a feeling of satisfaction from being able to accomplish more with less effort. Self-esteem and morale are bound to rise. In this sort of relaxed state, new ideas for solving old problems are likely to pop into your head while you walk. The calm solitude of walking gives you a chance to work things out in your mind as you move along. You can focus calmly on a current problem and its wisest solution. This is not likely to happen if you are sitting around worrying or mindlessly watching TV. Use those mental walks that we mentioned in Chapter 11.

## Walk Away Depression

Depression in our fast-paced society has become very prevalent. It may result in anything from a temporary dip in morale to suicide. It may be caused by personal misfortunes such as the loss of a loved one, chronic illness, ostracism by peers or any number of other causes at any age. In the young, many lives are destroyed before they have a chance to live if depression is allowed to escalate to intolerable levels. The common treatment is drugs—a temporary and artificial answer. We contend that exercise—brisk walking—should be the first prescription to try in combating depression.

The elderly are commonly afflicted with weakness, lack of mobility and lowered immune systems. The reason a good percentage of the elderly shuffle around and can barely walk is that their hips have atrophied through disuse to such an extent that they cannot move their legs more than a miniscule amount with each painful step. Whenever doctors see someone of advanced age who retains a great zest for living and has retained his vigor and self-esteem, they invariably find that person to be physically active in walking or some other self-propelled type of exercise. Plan ahead to be in that class.

## Too Much Rest Can Wear You Out

Fatigue can play a big part in our everyday lives, and it, along with insomnia and chronic tiredness, may or may not be a symptom of organic disease. Only your physician can tell for sure. However, most people are fatigued because of their sedentary lifestyle. Physical fatigue along with sleeplessness is often an indicator of lack of exercise. Ironically, the cure for fatigue and restlessness is not more rest but the right kind of aerobic exercise.

Does it seem odd to you that you can walk away from fatigue? You can! Physical, emotional, psychological and mental fatigues are all states in which you owe your body more oxygen than you are giving it. A highly trained endurance athlete can be physically exhausted at the end of a race. He used more energy than he was providing in his extended effort to maximize his performance. He equaled or exceeded the limits of his exertion capabilities. He does, however, recover very quickly and can even feel exhilarated a short time later because of his superb conditioning.

In contrast, a corporate executive can be fatigued after sitting all day at his desk, riding the elevator down to his car in the underground garage and heading home to flop on his couch. He did not even scratch the surface of his potential physical exertion level, yet he feels very tired, depressed and nervous. He doesn't know why he feels like this, but the fact is that his muscles did not supply him with enough oxygen to maintain the necessary minimum oxygen-consuming level for his body to function properly. He rests because he is tired and, as a result, he gets even more tired. In truth, such people are merely suffering from lack of one of the best things in life that is free—oxygen and the ability of the body to transport it to the vital organs. Our lungs were meant to be inflated, so we must breathe deeply and enjoy the benefits accrued from an oxygenated body.

## Don't Overdo Too Quickly

As much as we promote brisk walking, many among us are overachievers who think if a little of something is good for you, then a whole lot is bound to be better. People who jump into an exercise program with both feet and overdo are candidates for overstress. In order to manage excessive prolonged stress, you need to become familiar with its physical and psychological warning signs.

The following symptoms have been identified as signs of exercise overstress by that eminent researcher Dr. Hans Selye:

- nagging fatigue and general sluggishness that lingers from day to day;
- disinterest in normally exciting activities;
- low-level and persistent soreness and stiffness in muscles, joints and tendons;

• drops in performance level that are unexplained;

• excessive nervousness, depression, irritability, headaches, and inability to relax or sleep;

• diarrhea or constipation;

• frequent mild colds and sore throats;

• unexplained skin eruptions;

• aching stomach, possibly accompanied by loss of appetite and weight;

• swelling and aching in the lymph glands, particularly in the neck, underarm and groin areas.

Any of these symptoms, which are psychologically or medically distressing, can be the body and mind's ways of saying "ease off." When overstressing occurs, injuries are far more likely to happen. The best thing to remember is: Train—don't strain.

## Walk Away Anxiety

We contend that the most calming activity and best anxiety reduction measure is to take a walk on a quiet wooded trail away from the noise of madding crowds. Walk in a relaxed fashion and work into a comfortable pace. Think about breathing and body movements—blend them together into a comfortable synchrony. Take in and enjoy the beauty of the surroundings. Think about relaxing the various muscles of the body—the neck, shoulders, arms, hips, legs—one at a time until they are all in a loose state. As the body relaxes, turn all thoughts inward and think of pleasant things. Daydream a little. If you can learn to relax and meditate as you walk, you will find, after a certain amount of exercise, that the things that have been bothering you are not so bothersome anymore. Daydreaming should have the recognition it deserves as a therapeutic mind relaxer.

If the ability to relax through rhythmic exercise becomes well developed, the following benefits are likely to be realized:

• Thinking will be clearer.

• Need for tranquilizers and stimulants will be eliminated or greatly reduced.

• Work will be done more efficiently.

- There will be fewer headaches, high blood pressure and other health problems that often find their roots in tension and anxiety.

All indications point to the fact that a finely tuned walking program will give us the desired means to control the emotional storms that we all have from time to time. And all the side effects are very beneficial.

## CHAPTER 17

# REALISTIC EXPECTATIONS

*"Man, unlike any other thing organic or inorganic in the universe, grows beyond his work, walks up the stairs in his concepts, emerges ahead of his accomplishments."*

—John Steinbeck

---

We have made a lot of bold statements and claims of what our program can do for you. Now, you might ask, what is realistic? We think it is all realistic.

We know that most of you can add years of fun and productivity to your lives if only you will buckle down and work at it. Walk briskly every day for 45 minutes to an hour. Eat properly—a low fat diet (cut back especially on animal fats and simple sugars). Include a lot of fiber in your diet. Eliminate poisons such as tobacco, excessive alcohol (one glass of beer or wine before dinner is OK), unnecessary prescription medications, pills and illicit drugs. Basically, if you do these things in combination you can be a winner in the healthy lifestyle and fitness game. Then set some goals that will make you want to jump out of bed in the morning to get with it.

Some people think of their bodies as machines with parts that just naturally wear out with age. Wrong! Our bodies respond to physical stress by ADAPTING and growing stronger. Unlike machines, our bodies, instead of wearing out with use and getting weaker, get more vigorous. The more energy we expend the more we have to use! This response is what evolution and survival are all about. And this principle holds true for more than just muscles. For instance, our hearts and lungs don't get tired as we get older—they just get lazy. If you've been deliberately slowing down your pace to conserve energy, forget it. Make moderate physical demands on your body and it will respond with renewed energy. An experiment by a group of doctors at the Washington School of Medicine in St. Louis compared two groups of middle-aged men—a group of steady aerobic exercisers (average age 58) and a group of sedentary men. It turned out that the exercisers had roughly double the cardiovascular capacity of the sedentary group. Remember, the heart is just a muscle and must be exercised to be strong and well, like any other muscle.

## Set Goals Realistically

If you set your fitness goals too high, as if you were 20 years younger, you will get discouraged. Compare yourself with others of your own age, then you can see a real difference between yourself and your sedentary peers. It can be frustrating to try to completely turn back the clock, but you can feel a lot younger inside. Try to be the best and fittest of your age group no matter what age. That is a realistic goal.

Keep active both mentally and physically. There is no reason why you can't do all the things you think would be fun. The tougher things are just a bigger challenge, and challenge will keep you young and energetic.

How can we go about setting realistic goals? Let's start off with a list. What do you want out of life that you don't already have? If you could rub a magic lamp and be or do anything you wanted, what would those things be? What expectations of life haven't you yet achieved? All these things should go onto your list. Let the list run as long as your imagination will make it. Yes, we know we said REALISTIC expectations and goals, but you can't judge a goal realistic or unrealistic until you have thought about it seriously. Let the list be as fantastic as your wildest imagination can make it. Don't edit the list while you are making it. If a trip to the moon strikes your fancy, list it! Take a few days or even weeks to make your list. And feel free to add to it any time. Let your fancy fly.

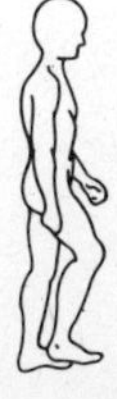

Recheck your list now and then, adding new ideas and scratching off the things that seem less alluring as time goes on. What remains is what you have to set down as realistic goals and expectations. Remember, what might seem out of reach for you today may not be at all out of reach tomorrow.

## Look to Tomorrow

If you are in your 50s now and you put the impossible task of climbing an 18,000-foot mountain on your list, then your first task is to make that impossible task possible. Maybe today you couldn't climb a 7,000-foot peak. Maybe today you are having trouble walking two miles with ease at sea level. Then your first subgoal is to walk those two miles with ease—then four miles, next six miles and so on. When you can walk eight to 10 miles, that 7,000-foot peak won't be much of a threat at all. And if you keep working at it you will make the 18,000-footer too. Maybe not in the shape you are in today, but in the great shape you will be in a year or two from now.

You set the limits. If you are not willing to work for it, you probably don't really want it badly enough. Go for it. If you don't get to the top of the 18,000-foot peak, you will be a better person for having tried, and if you make it only to 12,000 feet by the time you are 80 or 90, at least you will have headed for the top of the hill instead of the bottom.

It is those goals that will become the motivation to drive you on to becoming the new and better you. When you put something down on your list of goals and expectations, it is the wild fantasies that we want you to give the longest thought to. The point we're trying to make is: WHAT IS UNREALISTIC FOR YOU TODAY MAY BE A BREEZE FOR THE NEW YOU TOMORROW. What you are too weak and frail to do today, you can be strong enough to do tomorrow. What you don't have the skills and talent for today, you can train yourself to do tomorrow.

## Your Future Is Up to You

Remember, we don't want to just add years to your life; we want to add MIDDLE age years to your life. We want you to enjoy yourself to the recognized limit of human life—120 years or as close to it as you can get. We want you to celebrate the last day of your life by being able to take a long, brisk walk thinking about what you have planned for the next day. That is realistic—but only if you stick with an active program. Your future is up to you and you cannot put the responsibility on anyone else.

The alternative is to keep on a downhill course. Remember, downhill travel can be very swift, and all you will be hurrying to is a six-foot hole in the ground. Better to set your sights on the top of the hill. It may take a little more effort, but the rewards are a lot more gratifying.

People in their 60s, 70s, 80s and older can go to college, take music lessons and dancing lessons, learn to ski and even think about getting in shape to visit the moon. It can all start right now by taking a walk a little faster and farther than the one you took yesterday.

## CHAPTER 18

# STICKING WITH IT

*"Above all, do not lose your desire to walk: every day I walk myself into a state of well-being and walk away from every illness. I have walked myself into my best thoughts and I know of no thought so burdensome that I cannot walk away from it."*

—Kierkegaard

---

At times we have all been filled with the best intentions regarding our diets and our exercise programs, but some of us have slipped back and neglected both of these disciplines. Look into the mirror, monitor how you currently feel about your appearance and self-esteem. Do you see room for improvement? What do you need to do to keep from backsliding even farther? How do you keep it from happening again?

Perseverance is the key. We need to get it into our minds that we really must take charge of our lives. We must truly desire to live the "good life," filled with enough energy to do all the things we wish to do—including having fun. We must realize that life was not meant to be a spectator sport, that to be fulfilled we must all take an active part in things that make life challenging and satisfying.

What we recommend is a program of sensible eating and exercise habits that you can live with for the rest of your days. Small progressive changes can easily be tolerated, but drastic measures cannot most of the time. No one can live forever avoiding the foods he loves while trying to adhere to a fad diet that is supposed to knock off pounds daily. Eat in moderation and build up the exercise intensity gradually while being patient and persistent enough to reach your subgoals one at a time.

You can acquire a taste for nutritious foods if you start eating them more, and acquiring this taste should be one of your goals. You can diminish your desire for excess sweets and fats as you get into better and better shape. You will discover that highly nutritious foods give you far more energy, strength and endurance to do vigorous activities than do the empty-calorie sweets that cause an insulin reaction, and fatty meats that sit in your stomach for long periods of time before they digest. And remember that it is extremely counterproductive to lose weight too rapidly, as we discuss in Chapter 9, "Your Healthy Diet."

What is going to keep you working out and adhering to your new total lifestyle? If you have been at it for several weeks, you have already discovered that total fitness is its own reward. If your body is not hungering for increased physical activity, be assured that it soon will.

## Excuses . . . Excuses . . . Excuses

Again and again we hear the same excuses for not exercising. It seems that for some people, the threat of poor health or premature death is not enough of an incentive to opt for a good lifestyle with plenty of exercise. They know full well that carrying excess weight is causing a strain on their backs and hearts, that it increases high blood pressure and that lack of exercise increases their chances of heart attack or stroke. Some of the following clichés are included in the sedentary person's rebuttal to reminders of health risks:

1. It is no fun living unless I can eat and drink what I want, so I want to enjoy these things while I can.
2. I am basically healthy and seldom sick. I don't seem to need all that exercise and fitness.
3. I'll gain too much weight if I quit smoking.
4. I know some people who don't exercise and drink and smoke, and they still live to an old age.
5. I have to die of something—I might as well die of

something I enjoy such as smoking, drinking or getting stoned on drugs.

6. When my time comes I am going to die and there is nothing I can do about it.

7. I am so far out of shape now that I don't think my poor body could tolerate exercise without risking a heart attack.

8. The prospect of death is so depressing that I don't want to address the problem or even think about it.

9. I feel all right now and will wait until later in life when I really need the exercise.

## Enjoy the Rewards of Fitness

Isn't it great to realize that you have much more endurance than you had just a few weeks ago? Isn't it just great to know that in a few more weeks you will be in even better shape? To know that you are not going in the direction of sedentariness, as you may have been before you started your fitness program?

Go through the list of motives for getting into shape listed in the beginning of this book, then review those you listed in the previous chapter, and see where you are starting to fit in. Think about the good feeling you have every time you reach another of your subgoals. And then think about the old days and how you felt when someone commented on the growing paunch so common to middle-aged men or the widening hips that plague women. Didn't it irritate you to discard perfectly good clothes that became too small? Think about the fact that you will never need to suffer these indignities ever again as you get into excellent physical shape. Your weight will likely stabilize at a healthy level and there are numerous other rewards to be reaped.

Although walking has the lowest dropout rate of any major exercise in the United States, no exercise program is likely to be maintained unless it is enjoyable. If you follow our advice you can make it so. Strolling at very slow speeds can be enjoyable and good for mental health, but it does little to benefit physical health. To achieve the rewards of fitness you have to get into brisk walking. At first there may be some fatigue, muscle soreness and weary feet, but take heart—it doesn't take long to get to the point where it is pure joy to get out and stretch your legs and ventilate your lungs. Seek the support of your family members or friends, or ask them to join into the activity with you. Walking can be a very social and therefore pleasant activity when done with others.

Don't be discouraged when you reach "plateaus" where no appreciable progress seems to occur. This is entirely normal and is to be expected. Be assured that breakthroughs will follow. Even if you slip off your program and do gain a few pounds, isn't it reassuring to know that you don't need to go on a deprivation diet to get the weight back off? Just go back to eating sensibly and getting into a fitness/walking regimen.

## Motivation Is a Must

What should you do to keep your motivation up in your beginning stages of aerobic walking? First you can find ways to make it more convenient and enjoyable. Choose the most pleasant routes you can find, away from heavily traveled streets or roads. Most parks are excellent for walking, and trails through the woods can be full of natural discoveries and rewards. Determine the most logical time of day for your own particular situation and try to make it a habit to set aside 30 or more uninterrupted minutes for the activity.

Pay attention to your body. Learn to relax as you develop a rapid, fluid stride. Tight muscles tire easily, so relaxing them is important. Allow your body to unwind and flow through the movements. If you get too breathless, or if you have difficulty talking to your walking partner, it is time to slow down just a little until you are more comfortable.

Learn what your ideal pulse rate should be and try to keep it within that range. You will soon notice the difference between your working and resting heart rates.

Try to wear the right clothes for the weather conditions. Most people tend to overdress in cold weather. The fact is that the body produces a great amount of heat during exercise—more than most people realize. Use the layered approach so that you can take things off and tie them around your waist if you get too hot and sweaty. In cold, breezy weather a good windbreaker is an essential item for an outer garment.

Do not skimp on footwear! Do your best to find the most comfortable walking shoes you can. If your shoes are either too large or too small, blisters will likely result. Lightweight shoes, as long as they have good support in the arches and a firm heel counter, make walking more fun. Make sure that there is ample room in the toe box so that the toes are not cramped. There are plenty of walking shoes on the market that will fill the bill in this regard. Nothing is more of a disincentive to walking than aching or blistered feet. Proper foot care is vital to your enjoyment and success.

A great advantage to an aerobic walking program is that it will eventually get you in such good shape that you can participate in practically any other activity that you choose. In this way you can broaden your interests and make life more interesting. This is certainly a motivating influence.

Establish achievable goals in your walking program. Don't "bite off more than you can chew." Nothing is more discouraging than consistent failure. Goal setting, whether it is weight loss or anything else, is an important motivational tool. Unreasonably tough goals unattained, however, can cause a stressful situation. Flexibility in establishing your own personal goals can affect your success in obtaining real benefits. If you use a moderate approach, are patient and look only for gradual improvement (not immediate dramatic improvement), you are on the right track. There are peaks, valleys and plateaus; but overall gradual improvement is to be expected.

## Personal Commitment to Exercise

Even the busiest people can make time for exercise and fitness programs ranging from modest to rigorous. Good evidence of this is that two of Colorado's most dedicated local exercise and fitness buffs are former Governor Richard Lamm and Mayor Federico Peña of Denver. It would be hard to find people with more demanding schedules and time commitments than these two "jocks," yet somehow, almost every day, they find or MAKE the time to keep their bodies and souls together with rigorous aerobic training—even if it means getting up at 5 a.m.!

For our regimens we should plan ahead on our calendars from week to week and then stick to it unless it is made impossible by some emergency. It is easy for unexpected things to get in the way if this personal time is not blocked out. If you must cancel, make an effort to find another time. It is all too easy to let things slide by and soon get out of the habit altogether. Actually, exercise does not have to be cut out entirely in any case, because we all must do some walking every day. As long as the walk is done at a brisk pace, you will be getting good exercise. It is important that you get the support of family members and/or working associates and others who make requests for your time. Let them know that your personal health, fitness, strength and productivity are very important to you so that they will understand the time you take.

Even if you must start out with a modest walking program—do it! The most important thing is just to get started and get into action, no matter what. It is easy to build the intensity and duration gradually as you go along. Take a walking break during your lunch hour. Walk upstairs instead of using the elevator. Park a mile away from work and walk the remaining distance before and after work. These things take little time—yet are very beneficial. Just making time for exercise will be an effort well-spent and will give you an excellent return on your investment—with compound interest!

Here are some questions to ask yourself to help you better decide what your realistic goals for success should be:

1. What obstacles might deter me from realizing my health and fitness improvement goals, and how can I neutralize them?
2. Who among my family or close associates might help me in attaining my goal? Do I think I can get their support?
3. What is my personal assessment of my chances for success?
4. If I achieve my goal, what do I think will have been gained?

List ways and means that will help you start on your way toward your fitness walking goal, and do your absolute best to carry them out. Remember that you are only cheating yourself if you don't.

Remember that no one else but you can make the commitment to improve your health and well-being. You should realize that a workout is one-fourth perspiration (or physical exertion) and three-fourths determination (or self-discipline). In truth, the hardest part is just to get out and start moving. After that it is easy. It is a personal triumph over laziness and procrastination—a sign that you have taken charge of your own destiny. It is an investment in excellence. You can release an untapped reservoir of energy that you never knew you had.

The human body gets stronger and stronger as you use it more and more, which gives you a sure and excellent return for your investment of time and energy. If financial investments were as risk-free as this investment in your personal health, we could all be rich. Most of all, you will increase your self-esteem and feel much better about yourself, and all your friends and family members will notice this change in you.

Following our suggestions will not guarantee that you will remain motivated to be a fit and active walker for the rest of your life, but they should help. Intelligent management of mind and body should allow you to take charge of yourself, to be captain of your own ship and able to sail away into excellent health and fitness through brisk walking. We sincerely hope that we have given you the motivation and valid reasons for instituting a new and healthy lifestyle. In any case, the longer you stay with your fitness program the less chance there will be that you will ever get off it. Just keep going at it a day at a time—for the rest of your life—as you healthwalk to total wellness.

# USEFUL INFORMATION FOR WALKERS

## 1. Loosening and Flexibility Exercises

Although brisk walking is the best exercise there is for building a foundation for overall body fitness, you will find it beneficial to add to your flexibility and strength. There are a number of exercises that can add to your walking enjoyment by strengthening and loosening the walking muscles. The following exercises can be done at home or any other suitable place in 10 or 15 minutes per day and ideally should be done at least three times per week. Choose the exercises that you think you need the most for each session and vary your routine so that you get your whole body involved. Do not force the exercises by stretching too hard or doing them too rigorously at first until you become accustomed to them. Muscles must be stretched gradually lest they rebel and tighten with a rebounding effect. Gently and gradually are the key words of action. Let us warn those who are very stiff that flexibility exercises are best done *after* walking, when the muscles are warm from the exercise. For those people we recommend walking slowly until the body is warmed up, then doing the workout followed by a stretching session.

The following exercises are designed to be helpful in making your walking more pain free and pleasant:

#1 WALK WHILE WINDMILLING THE ARMS TO THE REAR.

This exercise is very good for loosening the shoulders and arms. It also helps with coordination between arms and legs for propulsion. Do for at least one minute.

#2 GRASP THE ANKLE BEHIND THE BACK WITH THE OPPOSITE HAND.

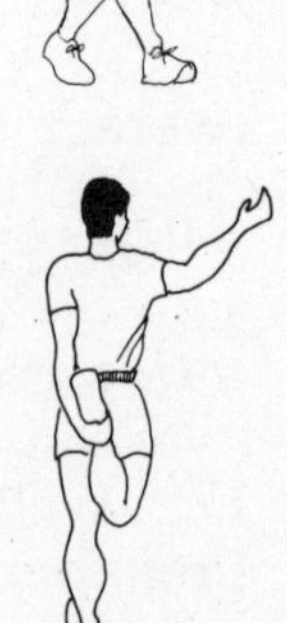

This exercise will stretch and loosen the knee joint and the quadriceps (front of thigh) muscle. Hold for 20 to 30 seconds and repeat several times for each leg.

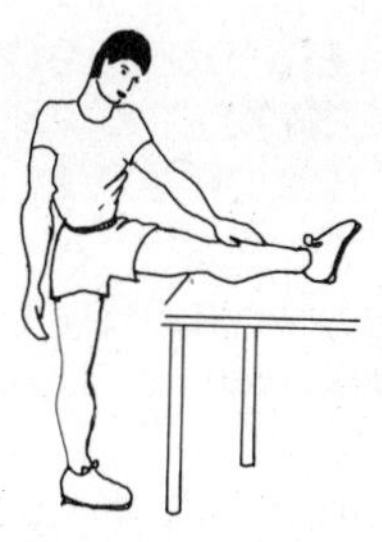

#3 PLACE ONE LEG ON A STATIONARY OBJECT OF AN APPROPRIATE HEIGHT AND GENTLY STRETCH. REACH OUT ARMS TOWARD TOES.

This will stretch the hamstring (back of thigh) muscle. Hold for 20 to 30 seconds and repeat several times for each leg.

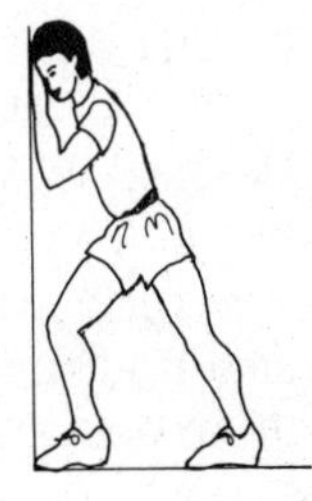

#4 PLACE FEET 24 to 36 INCHES FROM A WALL AND LEAN FORWARD. KEEP FEET FLAT ON FLOOR AND LEGS STRAIGHT. THEN ALTERNATE ONE LEG AT A TIME.

This will stretch the Achilles' tendon and calf muscles. Hold for 20 to 30 seconds and repeat several times.

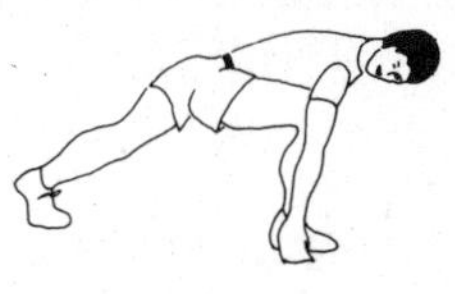

#5 SQUAT DOWN ON ONE LEG WITH OTHER LEG STRAIGHT TO THE REAR AND BOTH HANDS ON FLOOR.

This will stretch and loosen the groin. Hold for 15 to 20 seconds and repeat several times for each leg.

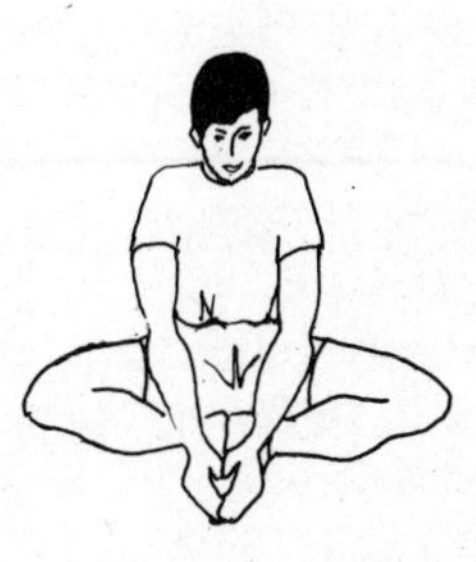

#6 SIT WITH KNEES BENT OUTWARD AND BOTTOMS OF FEET TOGETHER. GRASP ANKLES AND PULL UPPER BODY FORWARD.

Stretches the groin muscles. Hold for 15–20 seconds and repeat several times.

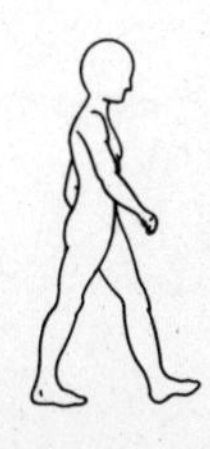

#7 LIE ON FLOOR ON SIDE WITH FEET HELD DOWN. RAISE UPPER BODY UP SIDEWAYS FROM WAIST.

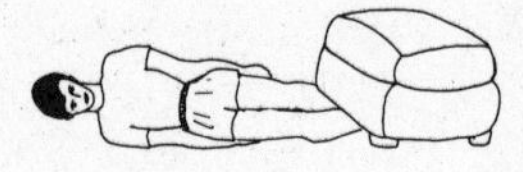

This strengthens the side muscles of the body. Repeat several times for each side.

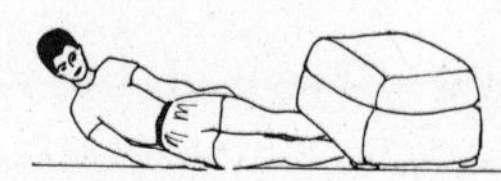

#8 STAND WITH TOES ON A 2- TO 3-INCH HIGH CURB OR OBJECT AND FLEX ANKLE UP AND DOWN.

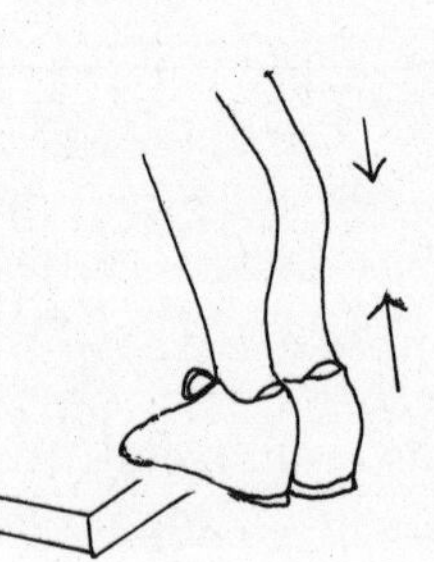

This flexes and strengthens the muscles in the shin area and the ankle joint. Repeat 20 to 30 times. (Particularly important for beginners.)

#9 WALK ON OUTER EDGES OF BOTH FEET.

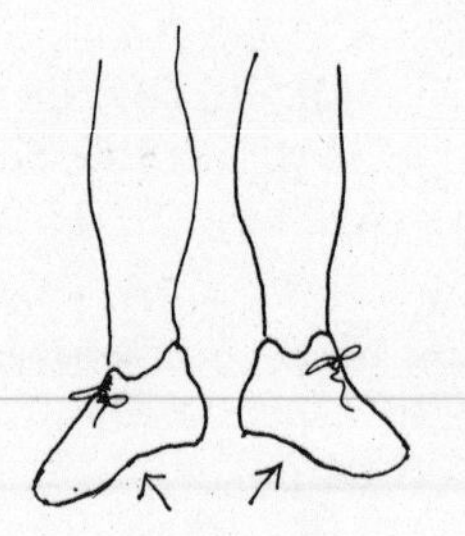

This strengthens the ankle and foot muscles which aid in foot push-off during the stride. Do until muscles tire and repeat several times with rest periods between.

#10 LIE FLAT ON BACK AND BRING ONE LEG OVER TO THE OPPOSITE SIDE. KEEP SHOULDERS AND ARMS FLAT ON FLOOR.

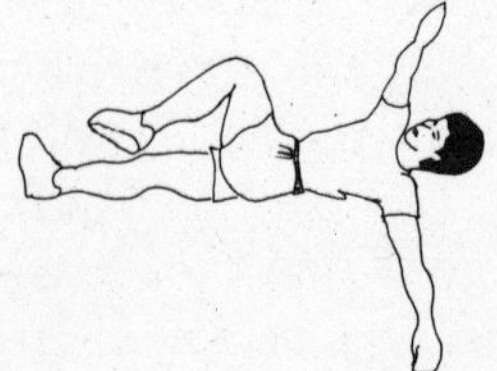

This stretches the hip and torso muscles. Hold for 20 to 30 seconds and repeat several times on each side.

#11 HOLD ON TO A POLE OR OTHER FIXED OBJECT AND STAND WITH STRAIGHT LEGS AS SHOWN. PUSH BACK AGAINST LEGS WITH ARMS.

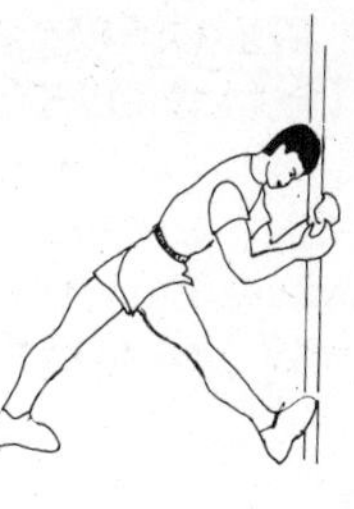

This increases the propulsive/pulling force of the legs. Hold for 15 to 20 seconds and repeat five times for each side.

#12 HOLD ON TO A POLE AND STAND ON ONE LEG WITH OTHER LEG RAISED HIGH TO THE REAR.

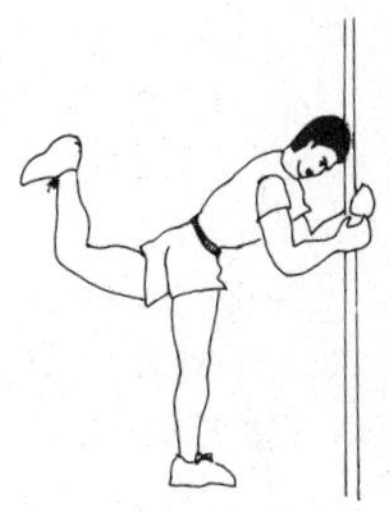

This strengthens the lower back and buttocks muscles. Hold for 15 to 20 seconds and repeat five times for each side.

#13 STAND IN PLACE ON STRAIGHT LEGS AND PUMP ARMS AND BEND KNEES ALTERNATELY AS IF WALKING.

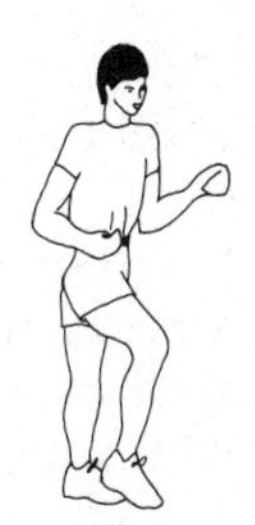

This coordinates the movements of brisk walking and promotes hip looseness and coordination.

#14 BOUNCE UP AND DOWN OFF THE FEET WHILE TWISTING THE HIPS AND ARMS FROM ONE SIDE TO THE OTHER.

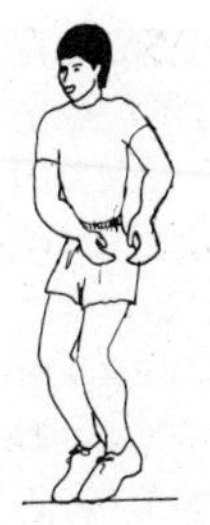

This is good for loosening the hips, stomach and diaphragm muscles. Do for 15 to 20 seconds and repeat several times.

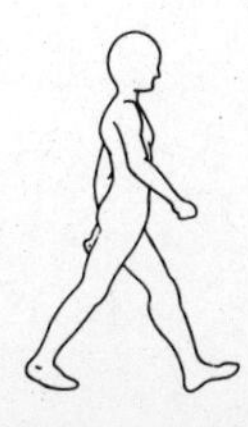

#15 RAISE TOES OFF THE GROUND AND WALK FORWARD ON THE HEELS.

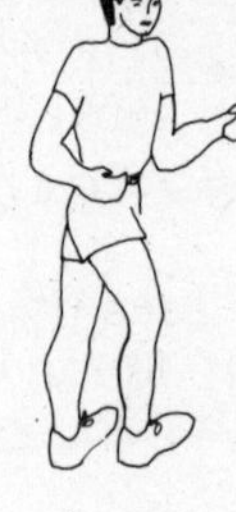

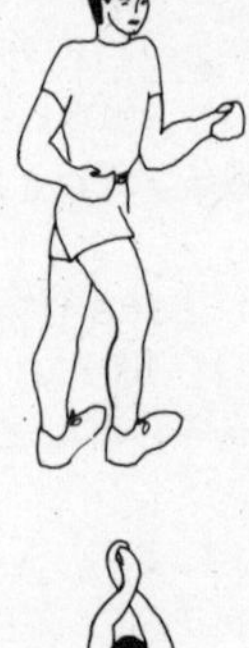

This is good for strengthening the calf and shin muscles. Do for 15 or 20 seconds and repeat several times with rest periods between.

#16 STAND WITH ARMS RAISED ABOVE THE HEAD, HANDS INTERTWINED.

This stretches and loosens the arms and shoulders. Hold for 15 to 20 seconds and repeat several times with rest periods between.

#17 STAND WITH FEET APART AND HANDS ON HIPS. BEND FORWARD AND ROTATE TRUNK AROUND IN CIRCLES.

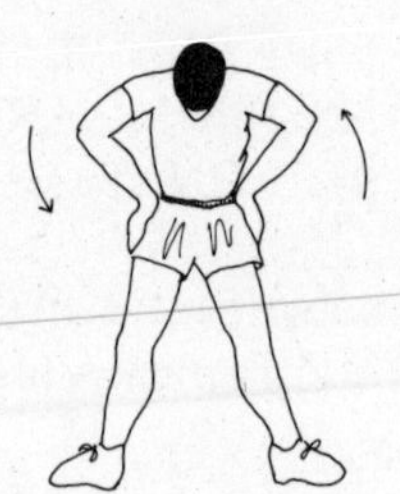

This is good for loosening hip, torso and abdominal muscles. Rotate 10 to 15 times.

#18 LIE ON SIDE AND RAISE STRAIGHT UPPER LEG REACHING UPPER HAND TOWARD LEG.

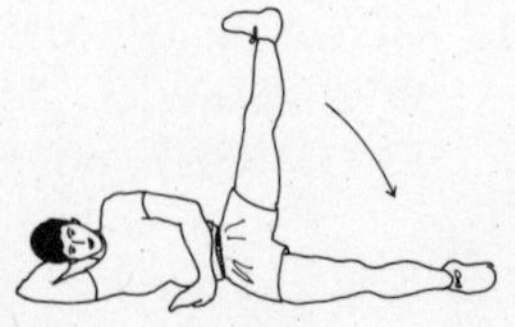

This is good for stretching and strengthening the torso and hip muscles. Hold for 10 seconds and repeat several times on each side.

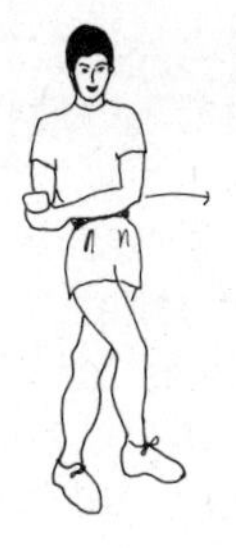

#19 WALK WITH HANDS CLASPED IN FRONT AND WALK WITH AN EXAGGERATED CROSS-OVER STEP WHILE SWINGING THE ARMS OPPOSITE TO THE HIP GIRDLE.

This gives added flexibility to the torso, shoulders and hips. Repeat on each side for 5 minutes.

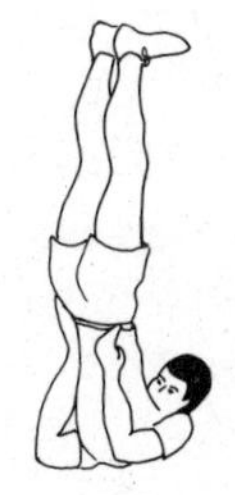

#20 LIE ON BACK AND RAISE BOTH LEGS ABOVE HEAD, SUPPORTING THE TORSO WITH THE ARMS.

This position is helpful to the lower back and buttocks. Hold for 10 seconds and repeat several times.

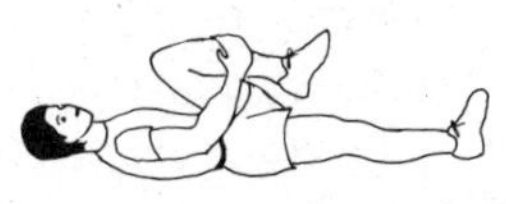

#21 LIE ON BACK AND DRAW ONE KNEE TO THE CHEST.

This position is good for the lower back and buttocks. Alternate, doing each leg for 10 seconds or more.

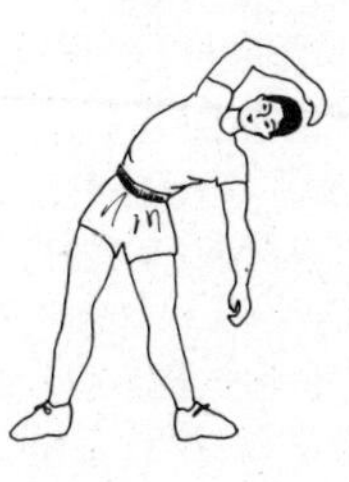

#22 STAND WITH FEET APART AND REACH TOWARD FOOT WITH SAME HAND. POINT TOE OUT.

This is good for stretching the muscles of the side of the torso. Hold for 10 seconds and alternate to each side several times.

#23 SIT ON FLOOR WITH FEET UNDER THE BUTTOCKS.

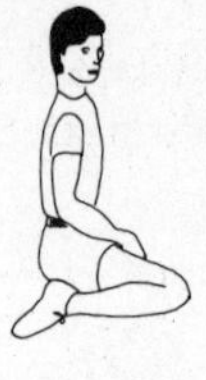

This is good for stretching the quadriceps (front of thigh) muscles and flexibility of the knee joint. May take some practice to reach this position. Hold for 15 to 20 seconds and repeat several times.

#24 SUPPORT YOURSELF OFF TWO TABLES OR THE BACKS OF TWO CHAIRS WITH THE TWO ARMS.

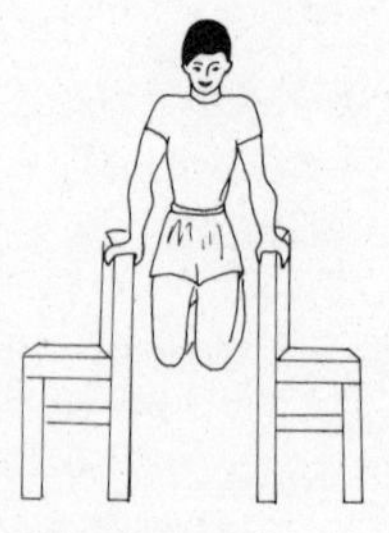

This is a good upper-body strengthening exercise. Try to hold position for 20 seconds or more. Increase the time as you get stronger.

#25 LIE ON BACK WITH LEGS BENT. RAISE UPPER BODY FROM FLOOR, USING THE ABDOMINAL MUSCLES. DO NOT GO MORE THAN HALF WAY UP.

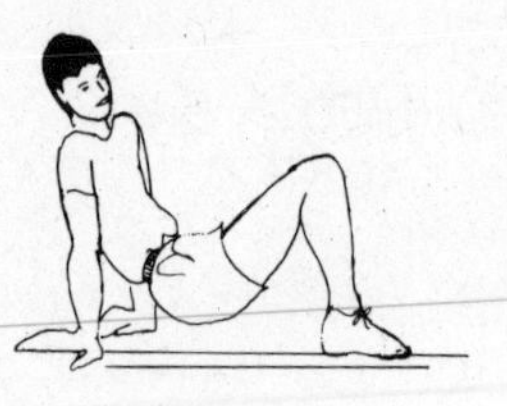

This is a very good strengthener for the abdominal muscles. Hold for a few seconds and repeat several times.

#26 FOLD ONE LEG UNDER THE BUTTOCK AND PUT OTHER STRAIGHT OUT IN FRONT. AS FLEXIBILITY INCREASES TRY TO BRING THE HEAD AND ARMS TOWARD THE FRONT FOOT.

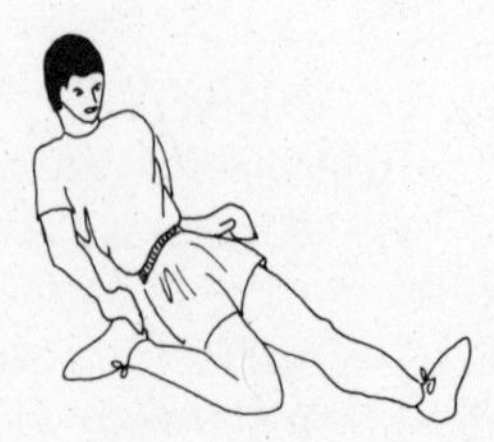

This is good for stretching both the front and rear thigh muscles (quadriceps and hamstrings.) Hold for a minute on each side and repeat several times.

#27 STAND AND LIFT KNEE TO INSIDE AND LOWER OPPOSITE ELBOW TO THAT KNEE. PLACE HANDS BEHIND NECK.

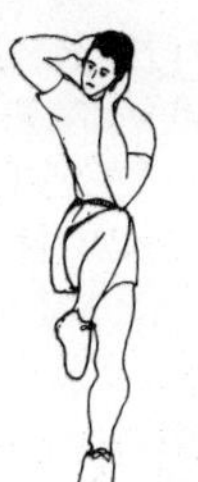

This is good for conditioning the waist and hip flexors. Do this as a dynamic exercise and alternate knees and elbows several times.

#28 STAND WITH STRAIGHT LEGS AND REACH BOTH HANDS TOWARD THE TOES.

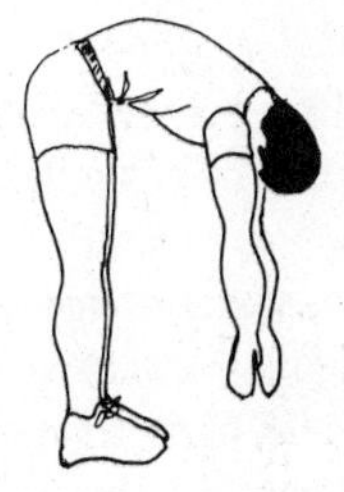

This is the classic exercise for stretching the rear of the legs and lower back. Keep legs straight and stretch as far as possible without straining. Let the stretch happen gradually.

#29 LIE FLAT ON BACK AND CURL NECK AND HEAD UP.

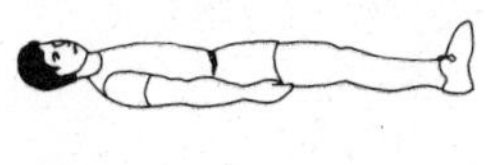

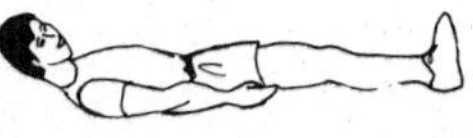

This is good for stretching and strengthening themuscles of the neck. Hold for a few seconds and repeat several times.

#30 STEP FORWARD ON ONE FOOT AND SWING ARMS AND TORSO IN THAT DIRECTION AS FAR AS POSSIBLE.

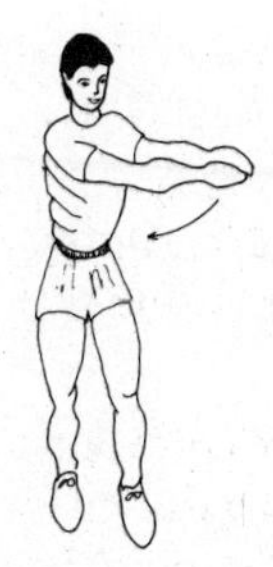

This is a good stretching exercise for the abdominal and lower back region. Exhale as body twists to the side and inhale as arms come to forward position. Repeat to each side several times.

#31 SITTING ON FLOOR, CROSS ONE LEG OVER THE OTHER WHICH IS STRAIGHT TO THE FRONT. TURN HEAD AND TORSO IN OPPOSITE DIRECTION. PUT ELBOW ON INSIDE OF OPPOSITE LEG.

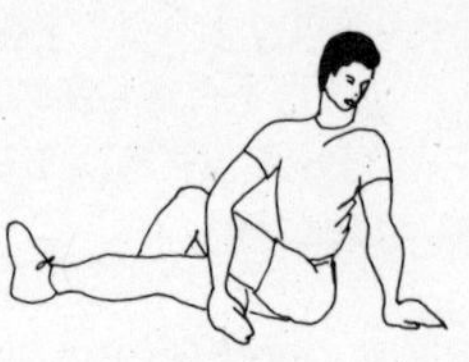

This stretches the spinal and torso muscles. Hold for a few seconds to each side and repeat several times.

The preceding exercises and stretching positions give a good selection of exercises and positions for strengthening and flexing all the muscles used in walking. There are many others to be found and you may even devise some of your own. Probably the ones that are hardest for you to do are the ones you need the most. Remember that strength and flexibility (along with endurance) are the things we must keep if we wish to remain or become active, supple and injury-free at any age.

*—Drawings by Suzan Polhemus*

## 2. Daily Training Log

You will find it helpful to keep a training log to measure your progress. This can be motivational if you are persistent in efforts to maintain your brisk walking consistently. You may find it interesting to estimate calories burned on each walk and keep track in the column provided. To do this use the following guidelines:

| Speed | Body Weight | Calories Burned/Hour |
|---|---|---|
| 3 mph | 100 lb | 210 |
| 4 1/2 mph | 100 lb | 295 |
| 3 mph | 150 lb | 320 |
| 4 1/2 mph | 150 lb | 440 |
| 3 mph | 200 lb | 450 |
| 4 1/2 mph | 200 lb | 600 |

If you walk only 1/2 hour, cut the values in half (or in proportion to your time). You may also interpolate as far as weight is concerned for an estimate—for example, if your weight is 175 pounds and you walk 4 1/2 mph, use a figure midway between 440 and 600 calories burned per hour, which equals 520.

**Sample Daily Training Log**
**(for photocopying)**

Date ______________________ Week Number ______________________

Your Goal ______________________ For miles walked this week ______________________

Resting pulse rate ______________________ Target pulse rate ______________________

Weight ______________________

| | Monday | Tuesday | Wednes. | Thursday | Friday | Saturday | Sunday |
|---|---|---|---|---|---|---|---|
| Weather conditions (temperature, wet, dry) | | | | | | | |
| Course (flat, hilly,surface) | | | | | | | |
| Pace (normal, slow, brisk) | | | | | | | |
| Target pulse rate (time maintained) | | | | | | | |

| | Monday | Tuesday | Wednes. | Thursday | Friday | Saturday | Sunday |
|---|---|---|---|---|---|---|---|
| Cool down (time and type) | | | | | | | |
| Duration of walk and estimated distance | | | | | | | |
| Est. calories burned | | | | | | | |
| Aches and pains | | | | | | | |
| How I felt (tired, peppy, relaxed, hungry) | | | | | | | |
| Days off | | | | | | | |

Notes and Comments ______________________________

## 3. Estimate Your Ideal Pulse Rate

(Average values to be used as rule of thumb)

| Age | Maximum Heart Rate | Maximum IPR 80% | Mid-Range IPR 70% | Minimum IPR 60% |
|---|---|---|---|---|
| 20 | 200 | 160 | 140 | 120 |
| 22 | 198 | 158 | 139 | 119 |
| 24 | 196 | 157 | 137 | 117 |
| 26 | 194 | 155 | 136 | 116 |
| 28 | 192 | 154 | 134 | 115 |
| 30 | 190 | 152 | 133 | 114 |
| 32 | 188 | 150 | 132 | 113 |
| 34 | 186 | 149 | 131 | 112 |
| 36 | 184 | 147 | 129 | 110 |
| 38 | 182 | 146 | 128 | 109 |
| 40 | 180 | 144 | 126 | 108 |
| 42 | 178 | 142 | 125 | 107 |
| 44 | 176 | 141 | 123 | 106 |
| 46 | 174 | 140 | 122 | 104 |
| 48 | 172 | 138 | 120 | 103 |
| 50 | 170 | 136 | 119 | 102 |
| 52 | 168 | 134 | 118 | 101 |
| 54 | 166 | 133 | 116 | 99 |
| 56 | 164 | 131 | 115 | 98 |
| 58 | 162 | 130 | 113 | 97 |
| 60 | 160 | 128 | 112 | 96 |
| 62 | 158 | 126 | 111 | 95 |
| 64 | 156 | 125 | 109 | 94 |
| 66 | 154 | 123 | 108 | 92 |
| 68 | 152 | 122 | 106 | 91 |
| 70 | 150 | 120 | 105 | 90 |
| 72 | 148 | 118 | 104 | 89 |
| 74 | 146 | 117 | 102 | 88 |
| 76 | 144 | 115 | 100 | 87 |
| 78 | 142 | 114 | 99 | 85 |
| 80 | 140 | 112 | 98 | 84 |

## 4. Figuring Distance Walked by Stride Length

Stride length is an important factor in walking speed and efficiency. The following table should give you a way to estimate distance walked by your natural stride length. You may wish to check the stride length at various speeds since speed does cause a variance. Check your stride when strolling comfortably—when walking at your minimum IPR (Ideal Pulse Rate)—medium IPR—and finally at your maximum IPR as defined in this section and in the text. Try to find a high school or college track of 400 meters or 440 yards. Almost all of the recent tracks are laid out as 400 meters, which is 2.6 yards short of 440 yards. Sixteen-hundred meters (a metric mile or four loops on a 400-meter track) is 10.2 yards short of a statute mile. This sort of accuracy is not too important for your purposes, but for long distances walked on a track the difference might become significant. If you want to take a relaxing walk to get your mind into action or to daydream a little, maybe going around and around on a track is the place to do it.

To establish your personal stride lengths, walk around the track counting your strides at various speeds, then you can determine lengths from the following table. With experience from your walking effort, you will soon be able to "sense" about what the stride length is when training or exercising, if you are walking on a fairly even and level surface. Then counting those steps will give you a fairly good approximation of each quarter mile (440 yards) or mile (1,760 yards) walked. If you happen to be where it has snowed an inch or two, you can measure the distance from one foot imprint to the other. Be warned that walking up or down steep gradients can throw your distance estimates off quite a bit unless you compensate for this. You usually take shorter steps going uphill and longer ones going downhill.

**Number of Steps**

| Stride length (inches) | per 400 meters | per 440 yards | per statute mile |
|---|---|---|---|
| 18 | 875 | 880 | 3,520 |
| 19 | 829 | 834 | 3,335 |
| 20 | 787 | 792 | 3,168 |
| 21 | 749 | 754 | 3,017 |
| 22 | 716 | 720 | 2,880 |
| 23 | 685 | 689 | 2,755 |
| 24 | 656 | 660 | 2,640 |
| 25 | 630 | 634 | 2,534 |
| 26 | 605 | 609 | 2,437 |
| 27 | 583 | 587 | 2,347 |
| 28 | 563 | 566 | 2,263 |
| 29 | 543 | 546 | 2,185 |
| 30 | 525 | 528 | 2,112 |
| 31 | 508 | 511 | 2,044 |
| 32 | 492 | 495 | 1,980 |
| 33 | 477 | 480 | 1,920 |
| 34 | 463 | 466 | 1,864 |
| 35 | 450 | 453 | 1,810 |
| 36 | 437 | 440 | 1,760 |
| 37 | 425 | 428 | 1,712 |
| 38 | 415 | 417 | 1,668 |
| 39 | 404 | 406 | 1,625 |
| 40 | 394 | 396 | 1,584 |
| 41 | 384 | 385 | 1,545 |
| 42 | 375 | 377 | 1,509 |
| 43 | 366 | 368 | 1,473 |
| 44 | 358 | 360 | 1,440 |
| 45 | 350 | 352 | 1,408 |
| 46 | 342 | 344 | 1,377 |
| 47 | 335 | 337 | 1,348 |
| 48 | 328 | 330 | 1,320 |

Through hip flexibility and rolling of those hips, stride length can be increased by up to 8 inches without perceived extra effort. The hip rotation then adds to the length of the leg in the stride. The added stride length, along with the quick reflexes to take rapid strides equal speed and efficiency. Extreme looseness in the hips is essential for both of these factors. That is how the elite racewalkers achieve the fantastic speeds that they do. As a point of interest, empirical experiments have shown that, for most people, walking speed is roughly two-thirds that of running speed for distances of a mile or more if you happen to be fairly efficient at both disciplines.

A non-hip-rotating, hiking style of walking is very speed limiting and causes the body to bob up and down, thus wasting some energy—you will be fighting a losing battle against efficiency and speed. However (using the above table) if you increase your stride length from 24 to 32 inches by gaining maximum mobility of the hips, you will be taking only 1,980 steps per mile as compared to 2,640. Since you have gained 8 inches on each stride (or .67 of a foot), you will be .67 (2,640 - 1,980) = .67 (660) or 440 feet or 147 yards or 1/12 mile farther than you would have been otherwise per mile. If you happen to be walking 10 kilometers in a race, it amounts to more than a half-mile advantage with no appreciable extra effort on your part. You can keep your stride frequency the same as well. That is why we stress that looseness and flexibility are not only the best ways to avoid injury, but help increase walking efficiency and enjoyment as well.

## 5. Assessing Chances of Developing Heart Disease

Relative Level of Risk

| RISK FACTOR | VERY LOW | LOW | MODERATE | HIGH | VERY HIGH |
|---|---|---|---|---|---|
| Blood Pressure | | | | | |
| Systolic | <110 | 120 | 130-140 | 150-160 | 170+ |
| Diastolic | < 70 | 76 | 82-88 | 94-100 | 105+ |
| Cigarettes (per day) | Never | 5 | 10-20 | 30-40 | 50+ |
| Cholesterol | <180 | 200 | 220-240 | 260-280 | 300+ |
| Triglycerides | < 80 | 100 | 150 | 200 | 300+ |
| Glucose | < 80 | 90 | 100-110 | 120-130 | 140+ |
| Body Fat (percentage) | | | | | |
| Men | 12 | 16 | 22 | 25 | 30+ |
| Women | 15 | 20 | 25 | 33 | 40+ |
| Stress-Tension | almost never | | occasional | frequent | nearly constant |
| Physical Endurance (walking at a rate of 4mph or more) | 4 hrs | 2-3 hrs | 1.5-2 hrs | 1/2-1 hr | under 1/2 hr |
| Family history of premature heart attack | 0 | 1 | 2 | 3 | 4 |
| Age | < 30 | 35 | 40 | 50 | 60+ |

## 6. Average U.S. Health and Fitness Standards

The tables below show how you can rate yourself in the health and fitness spectrum as related to your peers. Do keep in mind that the average figures for Americans are not very good, and you definitely should not be satisfied to be in this category. You should strive to approach the excellent category in all respects through your brisk walking program. Remember that for health, body fat percentage is a more important factor than absolute body weight. All heart rates are listed in beats per minute.

**Men—Excellent Health and Fitness**

| **Age** | **20-29** | **30-39** | **40-49** | **50-59** | **60 and over** |
|---|---|---|---|---|---|
| Maximum heart rate | 205-214 | 200-210 | 196-205 | 188-200 | 184-195 |
| Resting heart rate | 40-50 | 40-50 | 42-50 | 42-50 | 38-52 |
| Cholesterol (mg %) | 120-154 | 135-168 | 145-175 | 149-185 | 152-180 |
| Blood Pressure | 94–110<br>60 70 | 96–108<br>60 70 | 96–110<br>60 72 | 98–110<br>60 72 | 98–112<br>60 70 |
| Body fat percentage | 7.5%-11.5% | 7.1%-13.4% | 9.2%-14.9% | 9.0%-15.8% | 10.5%-14.1% |

**Women—Excellent Health and Fitness**

| Age | 20-29 | 30-39 | 40-49 | 50-59 | 60 and over |
|---|---|---|---|---|---|
| Maximum heart rate | 203-213 | 196-210 | 192-208 | 185-202 | 176-178 |
| Resting heart rate | 48-55 | 48-55 | 43-55 | 45-55 | 46-52 |
| Cholesterol (mg %) | 135-150 | 124-158 | 130-171 | 158-180 | 127-185 |
| Blood pressure | 90/58–100/63 | 90/60–100/65 | 90/58–100/65 | 90/58–108/69 | 110/66–120/70 |
| Body fat percentage | 4.8%-11.6% | 5.1%-13.1% | 7.3%-15.8% | 10.8%-18.2% | 6.8%-17.7% |

**Men—Good Health and Fitness**

| Age | 20-29 | 30-39 | 40-49 | 50-59 | 60 and over |
|---|---|---|---|---|---|
| Maximum heart rate | 199-200 | 194-198 | 188-191 | 180-183 | 170-175 |
| Resting heart rate | 40-50 | 40-50 | 42-50 | 42-50 | 38-52 |
| Cholesterol (mg %) | 165-178 | 182-193 | 193-204 | 201-211 | 196-206 |
| Blood Pressure | 112/72-118/78 | 110/74-116/78 | 111/76-118/80 | 116/78-120/80 | 120/76-124/80 |
| Body fat percentage | 13.9%-16.2% | 16.2%-18.2% | 17.7%-19.7% | 18.4%-20.4% | 17.2%-18.9% |

**Women—Good Health and Fitness**

| Age | 20-29 | 30-39 | 40-49 | 50-59 | 60 and over |
|---|---|---|---|---|---|
| Maximum heart rate | 194-198 | 192-198 | 183-186 | 176-180 | 160-165 |
| Resting heart rate | 59-60 | 58-62 | 60-62 | 60-61 | 57-60 |
| Cholesterol (mg %) | 165-170 | 168-176 | 184-195 | 198-205 | 210-223 |
| Blood pressure | 101/68-106/70 | 104/70-110/70 | 105/70-110/70 | 110/70-118/75 | 110/75-120/76 |
| Body fat percentage | 15.1%-18.3% | 16.7%-19.3% | 19.6%-21.9% | 22.7%-25.1% | 22.2%-25.1% |

**Men—Average Health and Fitness**

| Age | 20-29 | 30-39 | 40-49 | 50-59 | 60 and over |
|---|---|---|---|---|---|
| Maximum heart rate | 191-197 | 186-191 | 180-185 | 170-176 | 159-165 |
| Resting heart rate | 60-66 | 60-65 | 60-65 | 60-65 | 60-65 |
| Cholesterol (mg %) | 190-207 | 203-224 | 214-235 | 220-240 | 214-234 |
| Blood pressure | 120/80-128/80 | 120/80-124/81 | 120/80-126/84 | 122/80-130/86 | 130/80-140/84 |
| Body fat percentage | 18.0%-22.3% | 20.1%-22.6% | 21.5%-24.6% | 22.4%-25.0% | 20.5%-24.4% |

**Women—Average Health and Fitness**

| Age | 20-29 | 30-39 | 40-49 | 50-59 | 60 and over |
|---|---|---|---|---|---|
| Maximum heart rate | 186-190 | 182-185 | 173-180 | 167-173 | 150-156 |
| Resting heart rate | 63-70 | 65-70 | 65-70 | 64-69 | 62-66 |
| Cholesterol (mg %) | 182-196 | 188-204 | 201-217 | 218-234 | 235-245 |
| Blood pressure | 110/72-118/78 | 110/74-118/80 | 112/75-120/80 | 120/79-130/82 | 128/80-136/80 |
| Body fat percentage | 22.2%-26.2% | 21.5%-25.5% | 23.9%-27.5% | 27.0%-30.4% | 27.0%-30.8% |

**Men—Poor Health and Fitness**

| Age | 20-29 | 30-39 | 40-49 | 50-59 | 60 and over |
|---|---|---|---|---|---|
| Maximum heart rate | 183-188 | 180-183 | 171-176 | 160-166 | 145-152 |
| Resting heart rate | 70-72 | 68-72 | 69-72 | 68-72 | 68-72 |
| Cholesterol (mg %) | 218-229 | 238-250 | 245-257 | 250-264 | 250-264 |
| Blood pressure | 130/84-136/88 | 130/85-132/90 | 130/88-138/90 | 138/90-140/90 | 140/88-150/90 |
| Body fat percentage | 25.4%-28.6% | 25.5%-28.0% | 26.3%-28.5% | 27.0%-29.0% | 26.9%-28.9% |

**Women—Poor Health and Fitness**

| **Age** | **20-29** | **30-39** | **40-49** | **50-59** | **60 and over** |
|---|---|---|---|---|---|
| Maximum heart rate | 180-182 | 176-180 | 166-170 | 160-162 | 140-145 |
| Resting heart rate | 72-75 | 74-76 | 72-76 | 72-75 | 72-74 |
| Cholesterol (mg %) | 210-219 | 211-224 | 228-241 | 241-260 | 262-269 |
| Blood pressure | 120-130<br>80 88 | 120-130<br>80 88 | 120-130<br>80 88 | 134-140<br>85 92 | 140-148<br>86 94 |
| Body fat percentage | 28.2%-33.3% | 27.6%-31.3% | 29.1%-31.4% | 32.5%-34.7% | 31.7%-34.7% |

**Men—Very Poor Health and Fitness**

| **Age** | **20-29** | **30-39** | **40-49** | **50-59** | **60 and over** |
|---|---|---|---|---|---|
| Maximum heart rate | 179 or less | 174 or less | 164 or less | 150 or less | 131 or less |
| Resting heart rate | 80 or more | 77 or more | 78 or more | 77 or more | 77 or more |
| Cholesterol (mg %) | 251 or more | 271 or more | 275 or more | 285 or more | 280 or more |
| Blood pressure | 140<br>90<br>or higher | 142<br>94<br>or higher | 144<br>98<br>or higher | 150<br>100<br>or higher | 160<br>100<br>or higher |
| Body fat percentage | 32.8% or more | 33% or more | 33% or more | 33% or more | 33% or more |

**Women—Very Poor Health and Fitness**

| Age | 20-29 | 30-39 | 40-49 | 50-59 | 60 and over |
|---|---|---|---|---|---|
| Maximum heart rate | 172 or less | 170 or less | 158 or less | 152 or less | 126 or less |
| Resting heart rate | 84 or more | 84 or more | 82 or more | 84 or more | 80 or more |
| Cholesterol (mg %) | 251 or more | 240 or more | 264 or more | 275 or more | 280 or more |
| Blood pressure | 130/82 or higher | 134/90 or higher | 138/92 or higher | 148/92 or higher | 160/98 or higher |
| Body fat percentage | 38.5% or more | 38.7% or more | 37.4% or more | 39.7% or more | 36.9% or more |

## 7. Aches, Pains and First-Aid Measures

There are a few problems that might arise specifically from walking, but most can be avoided or reduced with a little thought and attention to preparation.

### Sprains and Strains

These are not as common among walkers as runners, but a twisted ankle might occasionally occur if you don't watch where you are walking. An overstretching and a tearing of a muscle, ligament or tendon may happen if you step in a hole or trip over a curb. Small blood vessels are broken and pain is caused when the surrounding area swells up and affects the adjacent nerve endings. These can be very painful, depending on their severity, and need to be rested until healed, or else aggravation of the injury is apt to occur. The biggest danger in this type injury is misdiagnosis of a simple fracture. It is therefore wise to get X-rays of all significant strains or sprains of a joint. Care to prevent further injury and expedite healing includes:

1. Remember the word RICE, meaning rest, ice, compression, elevation.
2. Do not bear weight on the injury.
3. For the first 24 hours after injury use cold packs to reduce the swelling. Avoid heat, which increases swelling.
4. Keep injured part elevated as much as possible.
5. If you must walk, use an elastic bandage wrapping for support.
6. Let a health professional examine the injury.

We repeat that prevention is better than first aid. A little forethought, planning and common sense will avert practically all walking injuries.

### Chest Pain

The most worrisome pains are those in the upper body and chest. These can be anything from inconsequential to serious—from being psychosomatic to angina pectoris. Most are not serious but should never be ignored, especially if they persist. The cause of pain may be merely heartburn or indigestion, which very closely mimics pains from the heart and is often relieved by an antacid. If the pain feels like pressure on the chest and subsides abruptly after cessation of exercise, the heart can be suspected, and medical advice should be sought. Even people who will never have a heart attack can experience the sensation of angina, since this is merely an insufficient supply of blood to the heart muscle. Psychosomatic or imaginary pain is often vague, but even so may cause similar symptoms of heart disease, such as palpitations, shortness of breath, exhaustion and chest pain. If the pain is not specific, it probably will test out to be negative by your physician. The mind and body are so closely intertwined that when we have an emotional event, we also have a physical one.

## Sciatica

Sciatica can cause as much misery as any ailment in existence. A sciatic-nerve injury can cause pain anywhere from the upper buttocks to the bottom of the foot—it can be anything from mild discomfort or a tingling to catastrophic pain. The main causes of sciatica are (1) structural weakness due to bony or ligamentous misalignments in the spine and (2) postural weakness caused by overdevelopment of the lower back muscles and relative weakness of the opposing stomach muscles. Walking has actually been used as a cure for runners who have developed a case of sciatica—especially racewalking, which in itself tends to strengthen the deficient muscles that cause the ailment.

Treatment should be aimed at flattening the spine and rotating the hips backward and the pubic bone forward. Bent-leg sit-ups are very good for sciatica. Other suggestions are to go without shoes at home to stretch the rear leg muscles. Sit with knees higher than the hips. Sleep on your "good" side with the painful side drawn up toward your chest. Avoid postures that cause lordosis or a hollow in the back (sway back). Chiropractic or osteopathic adjustments can provide temporary relief in many cases.

## Hip Pain

Hip pain is fairly common in the beginning stages of a walking program because there are previously little-used muscles being brought into play. These will disappear as the walker gets into better shape unless too much distance is covered too soon. Hip pain can come from a variety of sources—weak or high-arched feet, leg-length discrepancy, tight hamstrings, weak abdominals, overstriding; and going up and down too many hills. Hip-stretching exercises and bent-leg sit-ups are often very helpful in alleviating and preventing pains in the hip. Get sufficient rest after long walks so that the pain does not become chronic.

## Side Stitch

Beginning walkers will often get a pain in the upper abdomen, commonly on the right side. This is most often caused by a cramp of the diaphragm caused by pressure on it by the lungs from the top and contraction of the belly muscles from below. The cramp happens because of a lowered blood supply to the diaphragm. Cramping can also be caused by gas distending the colon. If the flow of gas is blocked by hard stools, the colon is stretched like a balloon, which causes the pain. It is prudent not to eat a lot of foods known to produce gas before exercising. Stitches are rare in experienced aerobic exercisers who are in good condition.

If a stitch occurs, breathe deeply using your stomach muscles and slow your pace. Often hard pressure with the fingers on the painful spot will relieve the pain. Bend forward and exhale hard while pursing your lips. Acupuncture books say to rub your fingers up and down on the center of your rib cage pressing vigorously to get relief. Probably the best preventive measure is to do exercises designed to strengthen the diaphragm and belly muscles such as bent-leg sit-ups.

## Cramps and Spasms

Cramps and spasms are a common occurrence. A muscle can contract powerfully and painfully—usually without warning—not only while walking but also in bed at night or at any other time. Causes can be dehydration, fatigue, cold weather, imbalance of salt and potassium levels, a sharp blow or overstretching of underused muscles. The occurrence of cramps can be reduced by eating a well-balanced diet with adequate salt and potassium, by drinking plenty of fluids, and by starting with a warm-up period or by walking slowly at first. Then stop walking before becoming overly fatigued. Cramps can usually be relieved by stretching or by a kneading massage of the affected muscle. Apply heat afterward to aid circulation. Try the "Loosening and Flexibility Exercises" in this section.

## Knee Pain

The knee is one of the most vulnerable parts of the body when a person is involved in weight-bearing exercises. Runner's knee, (chondromalacia patella) is a notorious ailment, and vastly more prevalent among runners and joggers than walkers. The knee is vulnerable because of a poor bone arrangement, and the fact that the main support is from tendons and ligaments. Knee-pain causes are almost always from the feet. It may be from walking on a slanted surface with one foot higher than the other. Weak arches or poor foot structure and improper foot plant are the most common causes of knee pain. If the foot collapses while walking, the lower leg rotates inward and the kneecap moves to the inside. Repeated foot strikes cause the kneecap to move back and forth and pain ensues. The knee may become increasingly irritated and swollen. Orthotics, professionally done by a podiatrist, may be the be best solution to correct the problem.

## Shin Soreness

Tenderness and pain in the shin area is often referred to as "shin splints." Causes may be a muscle imbalance from toeing the feet out, swelling of the muscle in the front of the leg causing a spasm or an inflamed tendon of the lower leg. The tendon may be torn from the bone, or there may be irritation of the membranes between the fibula and tibia or even a hairline fracture of the lower leg. Walking at faster than normal speeds often causes shin pain, because these muscles are seldom used otherwise. Wearing good footwear with a padded sole and avoiding walking on hard surfaces may alleviate shin pains. Exercises that flex the foot up and down, either with weights for resistance or lifting the whole body up and down are very helpful for this condition. Cold compresses can be of some benefit to reduce swelling and pain.

## Frostbite

Unless you live in an area of extreme cold, frostbite will be an unlikely problem for you. If you walk on very cold days, care must be taken to dress adequately and correctly. If you walk very briskly, you need not wear heavy clothing. The exercising body creates an amazing amount of internal heat. Several layers of thin materials will work better than a heavy one. Frostbite will most likely occur on areas of skin that are not protected from the cold air, or areas that are subjected to wet materials. Accordingly, make sure fingers, ears, and nose are covered with dry protection. Mittens are better than gloves for hand protection—some people even use heavy socks over the hands as a substitute for mittens. Simple ear bands can be enough to prevent frozen ears. Try to keep your shoes and socks as dry as possible. You may need to cut your walk short if your clothing becomes wet during freezing weather.

Recognizing frostbite is important since it occurs in small degrees. It may be manifest by a feeling of extreme coldness leading to numbness or tingling of the affected part. A bluish or ashen color may develop in the skin. If you even suspect the possibility of frostbite, begin the following first-aid measures:

1. Cover the affected area with a dry cloth, scarf, handkerchief or other protective material.

2. Get to a place where you can keep warm. Ingest a warm beverage or soup, but avoid alcoholic drinks. Alcohol causes vascular constriction and may further reduce circulation of blood which is necessary to restore the threatened tissue.

3. DO NOT RUB THE FROZEN PART. Frozen tissue is fragile and may be damaged by rubbing. Above all, don't follow that "old wives' tale" of rubbing the affected part with snow. This will only further injure the already hypothermic tissues.

4. Handle the frostbitten area with great care and gentleness.

5. DO NOT IMMERSE THE AFFECTED PART IN HOT WATER OR EXPOSE IT TO HIGH HEAT! Immersion should be into lukewarm water which can then be gradually but only slightly heated. The best thing is immersion in water around normal body temperature—97 to 99 degrees Fahrenheit. If in doubt, err on the side of coolness. If it is comfortably cool to your touch, it is an ideal temperature for use.

6. Go to the nearest emergency room or physician if severe, continuing first aid as you travel.

## Heat Exhaustion and Heatstroke

Perhaps the most dangerous weather for the walker is the hot, beautiful, blue-sky day with just enough breeze to keep you from realizing just how hot the sun is. It is this kind of day which can bring on heat exhaustion or potentially fatal heatstroke. For those walkers who are on salt-free diets, the danger might even be greater. We are more inclined to recommend curtailing your walking program on days of 90 degrees Fahrenheit and higher than on cold winter days. Caution must be exercised in hot weather. Walk in shaded areas if possible. Drink a lot of liquids—dehydration is the worst enemy. Carry water with you and drink more often than you think you need to. The feeling of thirst often has a delayed reaction. Salt tablets are of dubious value unless you are walking extremely long distances. Wear cool, loose-fitting clothing that will let air circulate around your body. In extreme conditions (either hot or cold) it is best not to exercise alone.

Symptoms of heat exhaustion or heat stroke include: weakness, lightheadedness, clammy to very hot-feeling skin, nausea, headache, extreme thirst, and faintness to unconsciousness. Symptoms such as these may occur in any combination or degree. If you suspect either heat exhaustion or heatstroke begin first aid as follows:

1. Get out of the sun and into a cool place as quickly as possible.
2. Recline on your back with your head elevated slightly.
3. Cool off with a cool damp cloth as quickly as possible.
4. Sip cool liquids but do not drink great quantities of liquid in too short a time as this may cause vomiting or choking.
5. Go to the nearest medical facility as quickly as possible and continue the cooling process during transportation.

## Blisters

The best prevention for blisters is good-fitting, dry equipment. Shoes and socks that breathe and move with your feet by holding them snugly will do the most to avoid blistering. Sometimes, even under the best of conditions, you might get a blister. First aid for blisters can be summed up in three words—KEEP THEM CLEAN! Soap and water are the best medicine and clean socks are the best dressing. Avoid cutting or picking the skin off of a blister until the tissue underneath has a chance to develop adequately. If there is any sign of infection—pus or extreme redness and heat—let your physician take care of it.

## Insect Bites and Scratches

Prevention is again the best remedy. Insect repellants are usually quite effective. If you are going to walk into possibly infested areas, make sure to spray some onto exposed skin. If you are bitten, keep the bites clean with soap and water. Most bites are not dangerous unless you are allergic. If you are extremely allergic you need to seek medical help. Some bites can get infected if you scratch them too much. Over-the-counter Benadryl taken either internally or topically can counter the itching effect.

If you get into scratchy plants or brush or slip and fall, scratches may result. Washing with soap and water is the best remedy. If any signs of infection follow (pus, redness or heat), get medical attention.

## Dog Bites

If this happens and the skin is broken, stop the bleeding with direct pressure to the injured area and get to a medical facility so that the wound can be properly cleaned. Even an insignificant-looking animal bite can cause severe infection (rarely rabies), so always err on the side of caution and get medical attention as soon as possible.

## 8. Racewalking History and Speed Records

It may come as a surprise to learn that racewalking has a long and rich tradition. Records show that walking races existed as far back as the 16th century. In the 1700s and 1800s walking races were held on a regular basis in Europe, including organized national championship events. Our famous American walker, Thomas Payson Weston, competed with and defeated the best in the world for many years. The sport was called "pedestrianism" or "go as you please" and the form was not judged. Many of the events were tests of endurance and included six-day events and others for hundreds and even thousands of miles. Wagering on the contestants was common to "add spice" to the contests. However, true racewalking, as we know it today, really began around the turn of this century with the return of the Olympic Games and the emergence of George Larner of England as walking maestro of the day and the father of modern racewalking technique. His style was universally regarded as flawless. Larner brought a degree of respectability to the sport, and it received official status with its inclusion in the 1908 Olympics and all succeeding Olympics, except in 1928 in Amsterdam.

In the early years, the Olympic events vied with ultra-long distance walks for popularity. Britain, the U.S. and Canada dominated early competitions, but the three-nation mastery was broken with the emergence of Italy's Ugo Frigerio, one of the most flamboyant and colorful characters in track and field history. Frigerio's crowd-pleasing antics included leading applause on his own behalf, giving lap-long fascist salutes to the crowd, trading comments with the spectators, etc. He brought a lot of attention to racewalking and won two Olympic gold medals in 1920 and one in 1924. Although his times fall short of today's standards, he clearly dominated his era.

Walking was dropped from the Olympics in 1928 but re-emerged in 1932 with the 50k event being contested. British walkers again rose to the top of the heap in the 1930s with occasional strong competition from the continent. During and after World War II, Swedish walkers were very dominant and some of their times would still be quite good today. The best of the dominating Swedes of that day were John Mikkaelsson and John Ljunggren. Mikkaelsson, with impeccable form, won the newly adopted 10k in the 1948 and 1952 Olympics, and Ljunggren won the 50k in 1948, 1956 and 1960 games.

Meanwhile during the forties, fifties and early sixties, U.S. racewalking sank to its lowest ebb ever with few real athletes in the sport—it was at the very bottom of the athletic barrel. A notable exception from this period was Henry Laskau, a German refugee and new citizen of the U.S., who competed quite well internationally in the forties and fifties. He now vigorously promotes the sport in Florida. Ron Zinn, who was killed in the Vietnam "police action," was a leading U.S. walker in the early sixties, and is now memorialized by awards given each year at Athletic Congress Conventions to outstanding competitors and promoters of racewalking.

In the sixties the Soviet Vladimir Golubnichiy emerged as the outstanding competitor in the world. He won Olympic gold medals in 1960 and 1968, bronze in 1964 and silver in 1972, all in the 20k (12.4 mile) event, which became the official distance for world championships along with the 50k (31 miles). He was dominant in the 20k worldwide for about 15 years. The U.S. had a breakthrough in the 1968 Olympic Games when Larry Young from Missouri won a bronze in Mexico City in the 50k, a feat he repeated in 1972 in Munich. Young's amazing accomplishments out of a relatively weak program, along with some outstanding results by Rudy Haluza and Ron Laird, gave impetus to the sport in the U.S. in the early seventies. Many of the present-day competitors have emerged from the New York state school system, which is about the only one in the U.S. that has had competitive racewalking. Women began competing in this country in the early seventies and their participation has been increasing ever since.

To enhance a racewalking program in Mexico, Jerzy Hausleber, an eminent Polish coach, was hired in the late sixties. Through his efforts competitors have achieved international success ever since. Such outstanding competitors and world record holders as Raul Gonzales (perhaps the world's best stylist), Ernesto Canto, Domingo Colon, Daniel Bautista and the latest sensation, young Carlos Mercenario (age 20 in 1987), have emerged from this excellent Mexican program. Our new generation of outstanding international competitors in the U.S. are Colorado's Marco Evoniuk, Carl Schueler, Tim Lewis and our best female, Maryanne Torrellas. With their renowned scientific training methods, the East Germans—especially Ronald Weigel and Hartwig Gauder—have also emerged as world leaders in recent years, particularly in the longer distances. Notable individuals such as Jozef Pribilinec of Czechoslovakia, José Marin of Spain and Maurizio Domilano of Italy have also won big events. On the female side, Kerry Saxby of Australia bears watching as a coming superstar of the sport. You may be amazed to read some of the following racewalking records. Many good recreational runners would be hard-pressed to *run* as fast:

**World Records—Outdoor Track (Men)**

| Distance | Time | Walker | Nation | Date Set |
|---|---|---|---|---|
| 1,500 m | 5:19.1 | David Smith | Australia | 8/11/82 |
| 1 mile | 5:45.15 | Martin Toporek | Austria | 9/11/82 |
| 3,000 m | 11:00.2 | Jozef Pribilinec | Czech. | 8/30/85 |
| 2 miles | 11:59.6 | Maurizio Damilano | Italy | 7/29/81 |
| 5,000 m | 18:42.0 | Jozef Pribilinec | Czech. | 8/30/85 |
| 5 miles | 31:23.1 | Maurizio Damilano | Italy | 8/22/82 |
| 10,000 m | 38:02.6 | Ronald Wiesner | E. Germany | 7/13/80 |
| 7 miles | 45:13.0 | Daniel Bautista | Mexico | 7/5/79 |
| 15,000 m | 58:22.4 | Jozef Pribilinec | Czech. | 9/6/86 |
| 10 miles | 1:05:07.6 | Domingo Colin | Mexico | 5/26/79 |
| 20,000 m | 1:18:40 | Ernesto Canto | Mexico | 5/5/84 |
| 15 miles | 1:42:18. | Reima Salonen | Finland | 9/1/79 |
| 25,000 m | 1:44:54 | Maurizio Damilano | Italy | 5/5/85 |
| 30,000 m | 2:06:07.3 | Maurizio Damilano | Italy | 5/5/85 |
| 20 miles | 2:22.1 | Raul Gonzales | Mexico | 5/19/78 |
| 35,000 m | 2:33:25 | Raul Gonzales | Mexico | 5/2/80 |
| 40,000 m | 2:55:54 | Raul Gonzales | Mexico | 5/2/80 |
| 25 miles | 2:57:02 | Raul Gonzales | Mexico | 5/25/79 |
| 30 miles | 3:34:17 | Raul Gonzales | Mexico | 5/25/79 |
| 50,000 m | 3:41:38.4 | Raul Gonzales | Mexico | 5/25/79 |
| 50 miles | 7:38:49. | Florimond Cornet | France | 6/25/39 |
| 100,000 m | 9:23:59 | Roger Quemener | France | 3/26/76 |
| 100 miles | 17:18:51 | Hector Nielson | England | 10/14/60 |
| 200,000 m | 22:16:40 | Hector Nelson | England | 10/14/60 |
| 1 hour | 15,477 m | Jozef Pribilinec | Czech. | 9/6/86 |
| 2 hours | 28,157 m | Jose Marin | Spain | 4/8/79 |
| 3 hours | 25 mi 739 yds | Raul Gonzales | Mexico | 5/25/79 |
| 12 hours | 73 mi 1584 yds | Ted Richardson | England | 10/16/38 |
| 24 hours | 133 mi 0 yds | Hector Nielson | England | 10/14/60 |

### World Indoor Track Records (men)

| Distance | Time | Walker | Nation | Date Set |
|---|---|---|---|---|
| 1,500 m | 5:13.5 | Tim Lewis | U.S. | 2/13/88 |
| 1 mile | 5:33.5 | Tim Lewis | U.S. | 2/788 |
| 3,000 m | 10.54.6 | Carlo Mattioli | Italy | 2/6/80 |
| 2 miles | 12.05.9 | Jim Heiring | U.S. | 2/28/86 |
| 5,000 m | 18:27.8 | Mikhail Schennilov | U.S.S.R. | 3/7/87 |
| 10,000 m | 38:31.4 | Werner Heyer | E. Germany | 1/12/80 |
| 15,000 m | 1:00.09 | Ronald Weigel | E. Germany | 1/27/80 |
| 20,000 m | 1:20.40 | Ronald Weigel | E. Germany | 1/27/80 |
| 1 hour | 14,906 m | Hartwig Gauder | E. Germany | 2/8/86 |

### World Road Records (men)

| Distance | Time | Walker | Nation | Date Set |
|---|---|---|---|---|
| 5,000 m | 18:29.0 | Josef Pribilinec | Czech. | 9/24/87 |
| 10,000 m | 38:48.8 | Josef Pribilinec | Czech. | 9/3/86 |
| 15,000 m | 59:43.0 | Josef Pribilinec | Czech. | 4/17/83 |
| | 59:43.0 | Jose Marin | Spain | 4/17/83 |
| 20,000 m | 1:19:12 | Axel Noack | E. Germany | 6/21/87 |
| 25,000 m | 1:45:52.0 | Hartwig Gauder | E. Germany | 7/20/80 |
| 30,000 m | 2:07:29.0 | Raul Gonzales | Mexico | 9/30/79 |
| 35,000 m | 2:30:43.0 | Raul Gonzales | Mexico | 9/30/79 |
| 40,000 m | 2:56:09.0 | Raul Gonzales | Mexico | 9/30/79 |
| 50,000 m | 3:38:17.0 | Ronald Weigel | E. Germany | 5/25/86 |
| 100,000 m | 9:07:00.0 | Zbigniew Klapa | Poland | 7/31/38 |
| 24 hours | 142 mi. 458 yds | Jesse Castaneda | U.S. | 9/18/76 |

### World Junior Record (men 19 and under)

| Distance | Time | Walker | Nation | Date Set |
|---|---|---|---|---|
| 10,000 m | 38:54.75 | Ralf Kowalski | E. Germany | 6/24/81 |

**World Records—Outdoor Track (women)**

| Distance | Time | Name | Nation | Date Set |
|---|---|---|---|---|
| 1,500 m | 6:03.3 | Kerry Saxby | Australia | 11/23/85 |
| 1 mile | 6:47.0 | Ann Jansson | Sweden | 7/5/85 |
| 3,000 m | 12:42.1 | Aleksandra Grigoryeva | U.S.S.R. | 6/22/86 |
| 2 miles | 14:00.0 | Giuliana Salce | Italy | 8/11/87 |
| 5,000 m | 20:55.8 | Kerry Saxby | Australia | 1/11/88 |
| 5 miles | 36.41.9 | Sue Cook | Australia | 9/14/83 |
| 10,000 m | 43:52 | Yaoling Chen | China | 10/24/87 |
| 15,000 m | 1:28:29 | Rosanne Feroldi | Italy | 10/18/86 |
| 20,000 m | 1:41:33 | Ann Jansson | Sweden | 10/25/87 |
| 25,000 m | 2:22.04.4 | Lucyne Rokitowska | Poland | 10/9/83 |
| 30,000 m | 2:56:36.0 | Cinzia Ghiandra | Italy | 10/18/86 |
| 35,000 m | 3:33:35.4 | Zofia Turnosz | Poland | 10/12/85 |
| 40,000 m | 4:06:21.8 | Zofia Turnosz | Poland | 10/12/85 |
| 50,000 m | 5:29:03.0 | Zofia Turnosz | Poland | 10/12/85 |
| 75,000 m | 8:42:46.0 | Beverly LaVeck | U.S. | 12/5/83 |
| 50 miles | 9:23:03.0 | Beverly LaVeck | U.S. | 12/5/83 |
| 100,000 m | 11:58:20 | Beverly LaVeck | U.S. | 12/5/83 |
| 150,000 m | 22:35:44 | Giuliana de Gobbi | Italy | 10/31/78 |
| 100 miles | 21:42.14 | Beverly LaVeck | U.S. | 12/5/83 |
| 200,000 m | 29:23.54 | Ann Sayer | England | 4/11/82 |
| 150 miles | 37:17.17 | Ann Sayer | England | 4/11/82 |
| 1 hour | 12,664 m | Giuliana Salce | Italy | 4/25/86 |
| 2 hours | 22,239 m | Jane Zarubova | Czech. | 10/12/85 |
| 3 hours | 18 mi 1559 yds | Lucyne Rokitowska | Poland | 10/9/83 |
| 24 hours | 116 mi 40 yds | Ann Sayer | England | 6/20/82 |

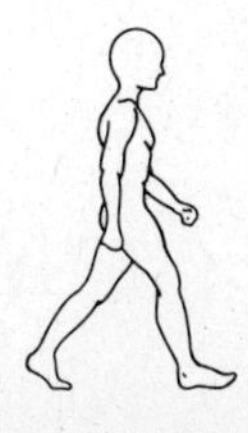

### World Indoor Track Records (women)

| Distance | Time | Walker | Nation | Date Set |
|---|---|---|---|---|
| 1,500 m | 6:01.16 | Maryanne Torrellas | U.S. | 2/14/87 |
| 1 mile | 6:28.46 | Giuliana Salce | Italy | 2/16/85 |
| 3,000 m | 12:05.5 | Olga Krishtop | U.S.S.R. | 3/6/87 |
| 2 miles | 14:49.1 | Sue Liers | U.S. | 2/8/81 |
| 5,000 m | 21:44.5 | Giuliana Salce | Italy | 2/20/85 |
| 10,000 40 yds | 50:52 | Andrea Werther | E. Germany | 2/8/86 |

### World Road Records (women)

| Distance | Time | Walker | Nation | Date Set |
|---|---|---|---|---|
| 5,000 m | 20:34 | Kerry Saxby | Australia | 9/24/87 |
| 10,000 m | 42:52 | Kerry Saxby | Australia | 7/19/87 |
| 15,000 m | 1:12.10 | Sue Cook | Australia | 12/19/82 |
| 20,000 m | 1:32:52 | Kerry Saxby | Australia | 6/14/87 |
| 25,000 m | 2:12:38 | Sue Cook | Australia | 6/20/81 |
| 30,000 m | 2:45.52 | Sue Cook | Australia | 9/5/82 |
| 35,000 m | 3:22.17 | Sue Liers | U.S. | 9/26/82 |
| 40,000 m | 3:52:24 | Sue Liers | U.S. | 9/26/82 |
| 50,000 m | 5:01.52 | Lillian Millen | England | 4/16/83 |
| 50 miles | 8:54:53 | Aaf de Rijk | Holland | 5/22/82 |
| 100,000 m | 11:40:07 | Aaf de Rijk | Holland | 10/17/81 |
| 100 miles | 18:28:01 | Aaf de Rijk | Holland | 5/22/82 |
| 200,000 m | 23:33:24 | Annie Meer-Timmermann | Holland | 4/10/82 |
| 24 hours | 124 mi 493 yds | Annie Meer-Timmermann | Holland | 4/10/82 |

### World Junior Record (women 19 and under)

| Distance | Time | Walker | Nation | Date Set |
|---|---|---|---|---|
| 5,000 m | 21:33.8 | Wang Yan | China | 3/8/86 |

## American Racewalking Records

### Outdoor Track (men)

| Distance | Time | Name | Date Set |
|---|---|---|---|
| 1,500 m | 5:39.0 | Ray Funkhouser | 8/5/84 |
| 1 mile | 6:09.9 | Ray Funkhouser | 7/6/85 |
| 3,000 m | 2:12.0 | Dave Romansky | 6/9/70 |
| 5,000 m | 20:01.9 | Jim Heiring | 5/6/84 |
| 10,000 m | 40:20.6 | Tim Lewis | 6/29/85 |
| 15,000 m | 1:02.34.0 | Marco Evoniuk | 5/5/84 |
| 20,000 m | 1:25:29.3 | Marco Evoniuk | 5/15/82 |
| | 1:25:29.3 | and Jim Heiring | 5/15/82 |
| 25,000 m | 1:54.43.8 | Ray Sharp | 12/23/82 |
| 30,000 m | 2:23.14.0 | Goetz Klopfer | 11/15/70 |
| 20 miles | 2:23.52.0 | Robert Kitchen | 3/21/71 |
| 35,000 m | 2:47.36.0 | Robert Kitchen | 11/21/71 |
| 40,000 m | 3:20:00.0 | Robert Kitchen | 2/27/72 |
| 50,000 m | 4:12:44.5 | Dan O'Connor | 11/18/83 |
| 100,000 m | 9:36:33 | Dan Pierce | 12/20/87 |
| 100 miles | 18:46:13 | Alan Price | 9/30/84 |
| 1 hour | 13,704 m | Neal Pyke | 10/15/78 |
| 2 hours | 26,131 m | Ray Sharp | 12/23/82 |

### American Indoor Records (men)

| Distance | Time | Name | Date Set |
|---|---|---|---|
| 1,500 m | 5:13.2 | Tim Lewis | 2/13/88 |
| 1 mile | 5:33.5 | Tim Lewis | 2/7/88 |
| 3,000 m | 11:16.3 | Ray Sharp | 2/3/84 |
| 2 miles | 12:05.94 | Jim Heiring | 2/28/86 |
| 3 miles | 19:40.0 | Todd Scully | 3/4/77 |
| 5,000 m | 19:18.4 | Tim Lewis | 3/7/87 |
| 10,000 m | 44:36.0 | John Knifton | 2/9/74 |

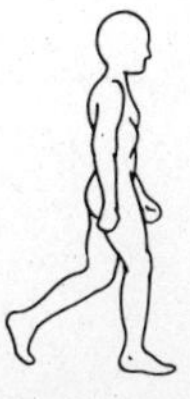

## American Road Records (men)

| Distance | Time | Name | Date Set |
|---|---|---|---|
| 5,000 m | 19:54.0 | Tim Lewis | 3/22/86 |
| 10,000 m | 42:15.0 | Marco Evoniuk | 8/21/82 |
| 15,000 m | 1:03:07 | Jim Heiring | 5/27/84 |
| 20,000 m | 1:21:48 | Tim Lewis | 10/5/86 |
| 25,000 m | 1:49:36 | Tim Lewis | 4/5/84 |
| 30,000 m | 2:16:41 | Marco Evoniuk | 3/19/83 |
| 35,000 m | 2:41:26 | Carl Schueler | 3/17/84 |
| 40,000 m | 3:13:57 | Carl Schueler | 9/23/84 |
| 50,000 m | 3:56:57 | Marco Evoniuk | 8/12/83 |

## American Junior Records—Outdoor Track (men 19 and under)

| Distance | Time | Name | Date Set |
|---|---|---|---|
| 3.000 m | 12:51.5 | Jim Mann | 7/6/83 |
| 5,000 m | 21:54.7 | Doug Fournier | 7/11/86 |
| 10,000 m | 44:20.8 | Doug Fournier | 7/18/86 |

## American Records—Outdoor Track (women)

| Distance | Time | Name | Date Set |
|---|---|---|---|
| 1,500 m | 6:46.6 | Lisa Metheny | 6/28/75 |
| 1 mile | 6:51.7 | Maryanne Torrellas | 7/9/63 |
| 3,000 m | 13:36.1 | Maryanne Torrellas | 7/6/83 |
| 5,000 m | 22:51.1 | Maryanne Torrellas | 6/29/85 |
| 10,000 m | 47:23.8 | Maryanne Torrellas | 6/20/87 |
| 15,000 m | 1:19:49.8 | Sue Liers | 3/20/77 |
| 20,000 m | 1:48:18.6 | Sue Liers | 3/20/77 |

## American Indoor Track Records (women)

| Distance | Time | Name | Date Set |
|---|---|---|---|
| 1,500 m | 6:01.16 | Maryanne Torrellas | 2/14/87 |
| 1 mile | 6:34.2 | Maryanne Torrellas | 2/19/88 |
| 3,000 m | 12:45.38 | Maryanne Torrellas | 2/26/88 |

### American Road Records (women)

| Distance | Time | Name | Date Set |
|---|---|---|---|
| 5,000 m | 22:57 | Maryanne Torrellas | 4/14/85 |
| 10,000 m | 46:28 | Maryanne Torrellas | 5/2/87 |
| 15,000 m | 1:13:39.9 | Debbi Lawrence | 2/7/87 |
| 20,000 m | 1:36.28 | Teresa Vaill | 11/22/87 |

### American Junior Records—Outdoor Track (women 19 and under)

| Distance | Time | Name | Date Set |
|---|---|---|---|
| 3,000 m | 14:35.38 | Lynn Weik | 6/21/85 |
| 5,000 m | 24:16.2 | Sue Brodock | 8/24/74 |

### All-American Standards for Masters Race Walkers

| Men | 5km | 10km | 20km |
|---|---|---|---|
| M40 | 24:30 | 51:00 | 1:45 |
| M45 | 26:00 | 54:00 | 1:52 |
| M50 | 27:30 | 57:00 | 1:58 |
| M55 | 29:00 | 1:00 | 2:04 |
| M60 | 30:30 | 1:03 | 2:10 |
| M65 | 32:00 | 1:06 | 2:16 |
| M70 | 34:00 | 1:10 | 2:24 |
| M75 | 36:00 | 1:14 | 2:32 |
| M80 | 38:00 | 1:18 | 2:40 |
| M85+ | 40:00 | 1:22 | 2:48 |

| Women | 5km | 10km | 20km |
|---|---|---|---|
| W40 | 29:00 | 1:00 | 2:04 |
| W45 | 31:00 | 1:04 | 2:12 |
| W50 | 33:00 | 1:08 | 2:20 |
| W55 | 35:00 | 1:12 | 2:28 |
| W60 | 38:00 | 1:18 | 2:28 |
| W65 | 41:00 | 1:24 | 2:52 |
| W70 | 44:00 | 1:30 | 3:04 |
| W75 | 47:00 | 1:36 | 3:16 |
| W80 | 50:00 | 1:42 | 3:28 |
| W85+ | 53:00 | 1:48 | 3:40 |

Those who meet these standards under judged conditions can apply for certificates from National Masters News, PO Box 2732, Van Nuys, CA 91404.

## 9. U.S. Walking Clubs and Prominent Promoters of Walking

**Alabama**
Ann Bibber
2301 Airport Boulevard
Mobile, AL 36606

**Alaska**
Lyle Perrigo
1921 Congress Circle #B
Anchorage, AK 99507

**Arizona**
Joe Kennedy
c/o AZAC Office
8436 E. Hubbell
Scottsdale, AZ 85257

Prescott Walkers
1150 Smokie
Prescott, AZ 86301

Gordon Wallace
102 Aztec Street
Prescott, AZ 86301

**Arkansas**
W. Randy Taylor
c/o Worthen Bank, Box 1681
Little Rock, AR 72203

**California**
Bauchet Street Walkers
c/o Ed Bouldin
9506 Pico Vista Road
Downey, CA 90240

Bob Bowman (IAAF Judge)
51 Chatsworth Court
Oakland, CA 94611

Brewer's Bullets c/o Bob Brewer
6811 Tahitian Circle
Yorba Linda, CA 92686

California Walkers
c/o John Kelly
1024 3rd Street
Santa Monica, CA 90403

Ron Daniel
1289 Balboa Court #149
Sunnyvale, CA 94086

Easy Striders Walking Club
c/o Jim Coots
2718 Monogram Avenue
Long Beach, CA 90815

Wayne Glusker
20351 Bollinger Road
Cupertino, CA 95014

Golden Gate Walkers
c/o Harry Siitonen
106 Sanchez Street #117
San Francisco, CA 94114

Myron "Tad" Godwin, Jr.
1811 Novato Boulevard #25
Novato, CA 94947

Robert A. Hickey
(IAAF judge, Teans, ISE/Coast Athletics)
9352 England Avenue
Westminster, CA 92683

Inland Empire Racewalkers
11878 Holly Street
Grand Terrace, CA 92324

Dr. Paula Kash
1124 1/2 Corning Street
Los Angeles, CA 90035

Lizzy Kemp
4350 Moraga Avenue #17
San Diego, CA 92117

Bill Langan
1472 Sierra Creek Way
San Jose, CA 95132

Lori Maynard (IAAF Judge)
2821 Kensington Road
Redwood City, CA 94061

Monterey Walk, Walk, Walk
c/o Giulio de Pietra
PO Box 221172
Carmel, CA 93922

North American
Racewalking Foundation
c/o Elaine Ward
1000 San Pasqual #35
Pasadena, CA 91106

Orange County Walkers
c/o Chris Rael
118 S. Pritchard #4
Fullerton, CA 92633

Saddleback Striders
c/o Barbara Sloate
24516 Sand Piper Lane
Dana Point, CA 92629

San Fernando Valley
Walkers (Women)
c/o Jim Bentley
PO Box 8120
Van Nuys, CA 91409

Santa Barbara Sport
Walkers Club
c/o Carell Jantzen
3791 Center Avenue
Santa Barbara, CA 93195

Roland Veon
128 Gold Canyon Drive
Ridgecrest, CA 93555

Walkers Club of Los Angeles
c/o Richard Oliver
11431 Sunshine Terrace
Studio City, CA 91604

Westlake Walkers
c/o Jim Hanley
3346 S. Allegheny Court
Westlake Village, CA 91361

Southern Cal Walkers
c/o Elaine Ward
1000 San Pasqual #35
Pasadena, CA 91106

**Colorado**
Jacques Adnet
4515 Diamondback Drive
Colorado Springs, CO 80908

Chris Amoroso
1815 Third Avenue
Longmont, CO 80501

Joe L Barrow, Jr.
675 Marion Street
Denver, CO 80218

Front Range Walkers
c/o Bob Carlson
2261 Glencoe Street
Denver, CO 80207

Lorraine Green
1015 Modred
Lafayette, CO 80026

Pamela Hahler
Gates Rubber Recreation
990 S. Broadway
Denver, CO 80209

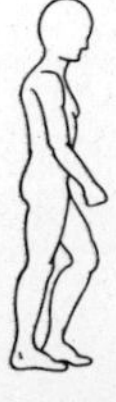

Leonard Jansen
c/o Olympic Training Center
(walking biomechanics)
1776 E. Boulder
Colorado Springs, CO 80909

Anne Kashiwa
c/o Oxford Athletic Club
1616 17th Street
Denver, CO 80202

Tim Lewis
(Olympic competitor)
326 1/2 E. Cache la Poudre
Colorado Springs, CO 80903

Paul Lightsey
2400 E. 16th Street
Greeley, CO 80631

Randy Mimm
1337 N. Tejon
Colorado Springs, CO 80903

Carl Schueler
(Olympic competitor)
326 1/2 E. Cache la Poudre
Colorado Springs, CO 80903

Viisha Sedlak
PO Box 18323
Boulder, CO 80308

**Connecticut**
Abraxas TC
c/o Rich and Maryanne Torrellas
28 Marion Lane
Clinton, CT 06413

Bruce L. Douglass
36 Canterbury Lane
Mystic, CT 06355

Bill Mongovan
12 Doubling Road
Greenwich, CT 06830

New York Masters Club
c/o Dr. Jack Boitano
Fairfield College
Fairfield, CT 06430-7524

**Delaware**
Rob Sweetgall
175 Elkton Road
Newark, DE 19711

**District of Columbia**
Bill Hillman
700 7th Street
Washington, DC 20024

**Florida**
Rex Cleveland
310 Murat Street
Tallahassee, FL 32304

Florida Walkers
c/o Bob Fine
4223 Palm Forest Drive North
Delray Beach, FL 33445

Dr. Terry O. Harville
279-10 Corry Village
Gainesville, FL 32603

Henry H. Laskau
(IAAF judge emeritus)
3232 Carambola Circle South
Coconut Creek, FL 33066

John MacLachlan
(Racewalking benefactor)
1330 Sable Palm Drive
Boca Raton, FL 33432

Dan Stanek
12123 Areaca
Wellington, FL 33414

Tampa Bay Walkers
c/o James McCarthy
12308 N. 27th Street
Tampa Bay, FL 33612

**Georgia**
Walkers Club of Georgia
c/o Dr. Bill Farrell
818 Peach Tree Center South
Atlanta, GA 30303

Dave Waddle
2327 Redfield Drive
Norcross, GA 30071

**Hawaii**
Debra Cottey
708 Hausten Street
Honolulu, HI 96826

Jim Moberly
415D Haleloa Place
Honolulu, HI 96821

**Idaho**
George Beall
2418 Elmcrest
Boise, ID 83705

**Illinois**
Augie Hirt
767 Bluff
Carol Stream, IL 60188

Chicago Walkers
111 W. Butterfield Road
Elmhurst, IL 60126

Chuck Klehm
1218 N. Route 47
Woodstock, IL 60098

**Indiana**
Sam Bell
Assembly Hall
Indiana University
Bloomington, IN 47401

Lee Rund
309 N. 25th Avenue
Beach Grove, IN 46107

**Iowa**
Ron Corey
133 West 3rd
Tama, IA 52339

Paul Schnieder
Siouxland YMCA
722 Nebraska Street
Sioux City, IA 51101

**Kansas**
Bari L. Garner-Holman
5728 Riley
Shawnee Mission, KS 66202

KC Walkers
c/o Don and Debbi Lawrence
4500 W. 107th Street
Overland Park, KS 66207

**Kentucky**
Willie Lewis
1304 Fairland Place
Louisville, KY 40211

**Louisiana**
New Orleans Walkers
c/o Richard Charles
4236 S. Roman Street
New Orleans, LA 70125

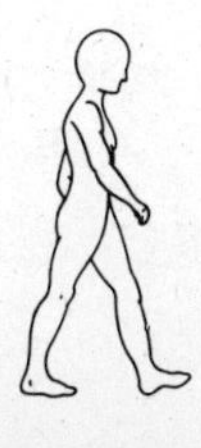

**Maine**
Larry Pelletier
19 Juniper Street
Bangor, ME 04401

Moshe Myerowitz
1570 Broadway
Bangor, ME 04401

**Massachusetts**
Betty Jenewin
Rec Office, Channing Street
Worcester, MA 01605

Tom Knatt
83 Riverside Avenue
Concord, MA 01742

Brian Savilonis
243 Mirick Road
Princeton, MA 02154

Steve Vaitones
90 Summit Street
Waltham, MA 02154

**Michigan**
Fabian Knizacki
Box 367
Ludlington, MI 49431

MCS c/o Jeannie Bocci
1353 Grayton
Grosse Point, MI 48230

Wolverine Pacers
c/o Frank Alongi (IAAF judge)
26530 Woodshire Avenue
Dearborn Heights, MI 48127

Frank Soby
3820 Harvard
Detroit, MI 48224

**Minnesota**
Craig Haugaard
Box 2013
Hutchinson, MN 55350

Bob Kitchen
917 5th Street
International Falls, MN 56649

**Missouri**
Columbia Track Club
c/o Joe Duncan
2980 Maple Bluff Drive
Columbia, MO 65201

Mark Young
6452 Smiley Street
St. Louis, MO 63139

**Nebraska**
Ruth White
3333 D Street
Lincoln, NE 68510

**Nevada**
Las Vegas Walkers
c/o Fraser Donel
Box 623
Mercury, NV 89023

**New Jersey**
Ray Funkhouser
1471 Arapahoe Court
Toms River, NJ 08753

Don Henry
24 Fairview Avenue
Bricktown, NJ 08724

Ron Kulik
10 Cleveland Avenue
Nutley, NJ 07110

Master Walker
c/o Alan Wood
Regency House, Room 254
Pompton Plains, NJ 07444

New Jersey Striders
c/o Ed Koch
PO Box 742
Madison, NJ 07940

Shore AC
c/o Elliott Denman
(IAAF judge)
28 N. Locust Avenue
West Long Branch, NJ 07764

**New Mexico**
Las Cruces Walkers
2025 Jordan
Las Cruces, NM 88001

New Mexico Racewalkers
c/o Gene Dix
2301 El Nido Court
Albuquerque, NM 87104

**New York**
Tom Edwards
67 Midland Avenue
Central Valley, NY 10917

Bill Gorman
1371 Kings Road
Schenectady, NY 12303

Island TC
c/o Gary Westerfield
(IAAF judge and RW coach)
Box 440
Smithtown, NY 11787

Dave Lawrence
90 Fairfield Avenue
Buffalo, NY 14223

Sue Liers
31 Cross Street
Smithtown, NY 11787

Bruce MacDonald (IAAF judge)
39 Fairview Avenue
Port Washington, NY 11050

Metropolitan Walkers
36 W. 20th Street
New York, NY 10011

New York Walkers Club
c/o Howie Jacobson
Box M
Livingston Manor, NY 12758

Dan O'Connor
2490 Woodland Avenue
Wantagh, NY 11793

Heliodoro Rico
Box 1504
Ansonia Station
New York, NY 10023

Dave Talcott
RD 3, Box 152A
Oswego, NY 13827

Walkers Club of America
c/o Howie Jacobson
Box M
Livingston Manor, NY 12758

Don Winiecki
61 Stewart Street
Buffalo, NY 14211

**North Carolina**
Eric Bigham
2511 Foxwood Drive
Chapel Hill, NC 28514

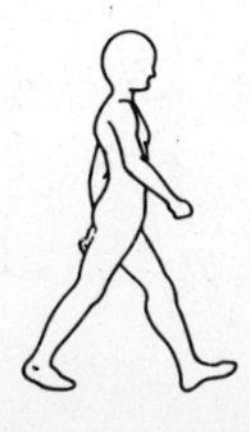

Southeastern Masters
PO Box 590
Raleigh, NC 27602

**North Dakota**
Shirley J. Olgeirson
PO Box 473
Bismark, ND 58502

**Ohio**
Edith Barrett
3801 Shannon Road
Cleveland Heights, OH 44118

Ron Laird
c/o 4706 Diane Drive
Ashtabula, OH 44004

Tim Melfi
PO Box 44
Dayton, OH 45428

Ohio Racewalker
c/o Jack Mortland
3184 Summit Street
Columbus, OH43202

John White
4865 Arthur Place
Columbus, OH 43220

**Oklahoma**
Loretta Hinkle
5312 N. Vermont
Oklahoma City, OK 73112

Oklahoma Fitness Walkers
c/o Ron Marlett
2712 NW 48
Oklahoma City, OK 73112

Tulsa Walkers
6764 S. 90th East Avenue
Tulsa, OK 74133

**Oregon**
Jim Bean
4658 Fuhrer Street NE
Salem, OR 97305

Oregon TC Masters
Box 10085
Eugene, OR 97440

**Pennsylvania**
Frank Greenberg
1414 PFFS Building
Philadelphia, PA 19107

Pat Mangan
570 Briarwood Avenue
Pittsburgh, PA 15228

William Norton
RD 1, Box 360A
Freemansville Road
Reading, PA 19607

Dr. Howard Palamarchuk
310 Middletown Boulevard #203
Langhome, PA 19047

Reading Track Club
112 S. Sterley Street
Shilington, PA 19607

**South Carolina**
Steve Sparrow
216 S. Edisto Avenue
Columbia, SC 29205

**South Dakota**
Bradley Knutson
811 University
Spearfish, SD 57783

Glen Peterson
1906 S. Hawthorne
Sioux Falls, SD 57105

**Tenneessee**
Hal Canfield
502 Alandale Road
Knoxville, TN 37920

Monte Towe
Box 59
Cookeville, TN 38503

**Texas**
Barbara Ayres
The Hills Fitness Center
809 Edgecliff Terrace
Austin, TX 78746

Tony Del Campo
3707 N. Stanton
El Paso, TX 79902

John Evans
5440 N. Braeswood #945
Houston, TX 77096

Dave Gwyn
6502 S. Briar Bayou
Houston, TX 77072

John Knifton
12900 Catskill Trail
Austin, TX 78750

Tom Lowry
4925 Matador
Amarillo, TX 79109

River City Walkers
2705 McCullough
Austin, TX 78703

**Utah**
Glen Wells
1963 Leisure Circle
Salt Lake City, UT 84118

**Virginia**
Potomac Valley Walkers
c/o Sal Corrallo
3466 Roberts Lane
North Arlington, VA 22207

Jean Wood
5302 Easton Drive
Springfield, VA 22131

**Washington**
Darlene Hickman (IAAF judge)
1960 Ninth Avenue West
Seattle, WA 98119

Dean Ingram
507 Cobb Building
Seattle, WA 98101

Pacific Pacers
c/o Bev LaVeck
6633 NE Windemere Road
Seattle, WA 98115

Lawrie and Gwen Robertson
14503 NE 65th
Redmond, WA 98052

Martin Rudow
(IAAF judge/RW Olympic coach)
4831 NE 44th
Seattle, WA 98105

Marge Snipes
2812 E. Hartson
Spokane, WA 99202

Ralph Varnaccia
Western Washington University
516 High Street
Bellingham, WA 98225

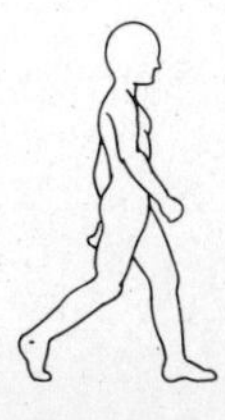

**West Virginia**
Nicholas Winowich
2003 Huber Road
Charleston, WV 25314

**Wisconsin**
BadgerWalkers
c/o Ruth Leff
6589 N. Crestwood Drive
Milwaukee, WI 53209

Mary Byers
6946 N. Shreve Avenue
Milwaukee, WI 53209

Mike Dewitt
814 40th Street
Kenosha, WI 53140

Larry K. Larson (IAAF judge)
909 Ostergard Avenue
Racine, WI 53406

**Wyoming**
Bernie Finch
Box 35
Newcastle, WY 82701

Clubs or promoters were not found for Maryland, Mississippi, Montana, New Hampshire, Rhode Island and Vermont. Please send information on these states to Bob Carlson, 2261 Glencoe Street, Denver, CO 80207. An IAAF judge is an international judge and considered to be a top racewalking official in the USA. This information is current as of 1988.

## 10. Starting a Walking Club

There are literally hundreds of running clubs in the United States at the present time but few walking clubs. If there is not a walking club in your immediate area, it may be enjoyable to start one yourself so that you can reap the joys of getting and staying in shape along with others of a like mind. If possible, assemble a group of four or more enthusiastic walkers who want to help establish a club. In our case we were able to assemble a list of more than one thousand names of people who were interested in walking—either fitness walking or racewalking. This was true mostly because a large corporation in Denver, Colorado, Wood Bros. Homes, and their marketing director Joe Louis Barrow, Jr., joined forces with the American Lung Association of Colorado in putting on walking clinics and low-key races at 5 kilometers (3.1 miles) in length, as well as a national 5k racewalking championship. Subsequently we were able to induct more than 300 paying members in about 23 months into our new Front Range Walkers Club. Eugene and Audrey Dix of New Mexico have also had good success in putting together an active club—the New Mexico Walkers and Striders Association. In another neighboring state, Ron Marlett has recruited large numbers for the Oklahoma Fitness Walkers.

Take the challenge and initiative and it can be done. Active clubs make the activity more of a social and learning event, thus more enjoyable for everyone. If you live in an area with few potential walkers in the immediate future, because walking hasn't received its deserved publicity, you may be better off persuading the local running club to add a walking division. This increases their overall membership and allows the use of their already established visibility, newsletter and equipment to get you off the ground. When the sport becomes more visible after a year or two, you can split off and set up a viable, separate club of your own. A catchy name for the club will draw people interested in walking. The term "racewalking" in the club title should be either downplayed or avoided because it is often intimidating to health/fitness walkers. However, we are not etching that in stone because in the near future the sport will be as popular as jogging or any of the other popular aerobic sports.

As in all clubs of this type, it is the small core of officers that make the club go. Dedicated organizers should divide up the duties according to their interests and abilities. Some of the things to be addressed are membership, promotion, finances, publicity, training and instruction, events (social and athletic) phone trees, newsletters and secretarial duties. The publicity chairperson is probably most responsible for a club's success—the word must be disseminated so people know about the club. The club will succeed only if the organizers put in the necessary initial energy to get it going. When the club becomes more recognizable, volunteer help will likely become more available.

To get members, go after all ages. It is fine to have a few competitive athletes, but the bulk of the club should be built around fitness walkers who are in it for the enjoyment of it all. And remember that walking is potentially the best family-oriented sport there is—the 80-year-old great-grandfather can have a ball walking with his 6-year-old great-grandchild—that is, if the elder of the two has embraced an active physical life. Look for runners who may have become hurt but don't want to lose their conditioning. Put out flyers in athletic clubs, schools, recreation centers and YMCAs as well as parks, libraries and athletic shoe stores. Print schedules of upcoming events and put them in the local newspapers. Make a concentrated effort to get your events listed along with the running events in the local newspaper and athletic publication (if one is published locally) and place low-cost classified ads if feasible. Have cards printed with pertinent information to be handed out to possible members. Talk race directors and/or sponsors into scheduling walking divisions in their races to add to the field.

To get the word out, set up free periodic workouts and instructional clinics at scheduled times and locations. Free instructional clinics will usually draw a few interested parties to the event if they know about it. Look for a central location around town to make events convenient for as many as possible. High school tracks and parks make good meeting locations. If you see someone walking briskly, approach them and tell them about your new organization.

Large shopping malls can be useful in regions with extreme climatic conditions. If you live in a cold climate, they may allow indoor fitness walks during inclement winter weather. Or take advantage of the air conditioning in the hot climates in summer. Retailers like to get as much traffic as possible into the malls because a certain percentage will buy something. Provide a real public service by offering to take in cardiac rehabilitation patients and recovering alcoholics from the local AA as members.

The club will need some operating funds to keep going. Charge a reasonable amount for yearly membership dues, such as $10 per year per individual and $15 per family. Try to play up the family aspect of the activity. Unfortunately the dues money may not pay for all the mailings and newsletters and incidental expenses. Ideally a sponsor will be found—many times new members that you enroll have excellent contacts with businesses, etc. Make some good club T-shirts and sell them at one or two dollars per shirt for a nominal profit. Charge race directors a fee for including a copy of their upcoming race blanks in your newsletter. Put a business' name on your T-shirt, if it donates the cost of them. Have a contest to find the best club logo to put on the shirts and newsletter. Some clubs assemble donated items and have raffles and yard sales. Accept healthy advertising in the newsletter. Charge for competitive events and pump the profits into the club treasury. Set up a walk series open to the general public and give each finisher a ribbon or some other low-cost recognition award such as a certificate with their name and time. Charge an entry fee about twice the cost of the individual awards.

Exchange newsletters with other clubs throughout the country (see our list of these in this section). You will get a lot of helpful hints and ideas from doing this and thus make your club more interesting to the members. Work for steady attendance at workouts. Have a calling committee that can set up a phone tree to contact members—that way each person may have to call only ten members or so. You will find that older persons and single persons will have more time to attend regularly because of fewer family and business commitments. Always encourage new members no matter how out of shape or non-athletic they may seem in the beginning. We have seen remarkable improvements in just a few months by people who have been motivated enough to stick to a steady program. Stress personal fitness and tell everyone at workouts how to measure their progress as time goes by (pulse rate, body fat, etc). As for competition, it is often best to have a handicap series in which contestants race against their own ability and speed standards. The slower contestants are given the appropriate head start based on previous times. The winner will be the one who does the best against his own handicap. Or you can have a predict event where the one coming closest to their predicted time is the winner. (No watches allowed in this event.)

Use some of these same principles to set up a club at your work site. Many companies all across the country are now organizing company clubs that get out and walk during the lunch hour and after work. We have seen some companies absorb the cost and make it entirely free for employees. They are realizing that such an activity is a benefit for both the employee and the company.

Walkers, in our experience, seem to share more of a comradeship and a closeness than in almost any other activity that we can name. We often marvel at the extent that this is so. Perhaps it is not as competitive as running and certain other sports, and everybody seems to want all the others to improve just as they have done. It is truly a family-oriented activity. Capitalize on this by having noncompetitive social events from time, to time such as potlucks and picnics so that the fast walkers have a chance to mingle with the slower ones and get better acquainted.

Stress the good fellowship and leave the highly competitive efforts to the few dedicated athletes in the club. Use the athletes as role models to show that most people can get in really good shape if they will persist in their efforts to improve. Most of all, don't be afraid to jump in with both feet and use a lot of energy to get the club going. As time goes by and your membership grows, more and more members will recommend the club to their friends and a "snowballing effect" will occur. A successful club is the source of a great amount of satisfaction, and you will be doing a lot of good in promoting health awareness in your community.

## A Bibliography of Interesting Walking and Health Books

Alongi, Frank. *Introduction to Racewalking.* Order directly from author: 26530 Woodshire, Dearborn Heights, Michigan 48127. $5 pb.

Bowman, Bob. *U. S. Racewalk Handbook.* c/o The Athletics Congress, Box 120, Indianapolis, Indiana 46206. (Published yearly).

Carlson, Bob and O.J. Seiden, M.D. *HealthWalk.* Golden, Colorado: Fulcrum, Inc. 1988. $12.95 pb.

Dix, Gene. *Racewalking and Fitness Walking Manual.* 1985, Order directly from author: 2301 El Nido Court NW, Albuquerque, New Mexico 87104. $7 pb.

Dreyfack, Raymond. *The Complete Book of Walking.* Arco Publishing Inc., 1981. $5.95 pb.

Fletcher, Colin. *The Complete Walker III.* New York: Alfred Knopf, 1985. $12.95 pb.

Gray, John. *Racewalking for Fun and Fitness.* New Jersey: Prentice-Hall, 1985. $16.95 hb, $7.95 pb.

Hopkins, Julian. *Racewalking.* Wimsey House, Box 33182, Granada Hills, California 91344. $6.95 pb.

Jacobson, Howard. *Racewalk to Fitness.* New York: Simon & Schuster, 1980. Order directly from author: Box M, Livingston Manor, New York 12758. $9.95 pb.

Kashiwa, Anne and James Rippe, M.D. *Fitness Walking for Women.* Boston: Raben Publishing Co., 1987. $9.95 pb.

Kiesling, Stephen and E.C. Frederick. *Walk On: A Tool Kit for Building Your Own Walking Fitness Program.* Emmaus, Pennsylvania: Rodale Press Inc., 1986. $7.95 pb.

Kuntzleman, Charles T. *The Complete Book of Walking.* New York: Simon & Schuster, 1978. $10 hb, $3.50 pb.

Marchetti, Al, M.D. *Dr Marchetti's Walking Book.* New York: Stein & Day, 1979. $4.95 pb.

Meyers, Casey. *Aerobic Walking.* New York: Vintage. $7.95 pb.

*Ohio Racewalker.* Edited by Jack Mortland. (Monthly newsletter with worldwide racewalking news and articles.) 3184 Summit Street, Columbus, Ohio 43202. $5 per year.

Pleas, John, Ph.D. *Walking.* W.W. Norton. $12.95 pb.

*Racewalking Judging Handbook.* c/o The Athletics Congress, Box 120, Indianapolis, Indiana 46206. $4 pb.

Ralston, Jeannie. *Walking for the Health of It.* Glenview, Illinois: American Association of Retired Persons, Scott Foresman and Co., 1986. $6.95 pb.

Reeves, Steve. *Power Walking.* Bobbs Merrill, 1982. $8.95 pb.

Rowen, Lillian and D.S. Laiken. *Speedwalking: The Exercise Alternative.* New York: G. P. Putnam & Sons, 1980.

Rudow, Martin. *Advanced Racewalking.* Technique Productions, 4831 NE 44th, Seattle, Washington, 98105. 1987.$9.95 pb.

Seiden, Othniel, M.D. *Walk—Get in Shape the Easy Way.* Blue Ridge Summit, Pennsylvania: TAB Books Inc., 1985. $6.95 pb.

Stutman, Fred A., M.D. *Walk, Don't Die.* Medical Manor Books. $9.95 pb.

——— *Walk—Don't Run—Stay Fit Without Killing Yourself.* Medical Manor Books, 1984. $8.95 pb.

Sussman, Aaron and Ruth Goode. *The Magic of Walking.* New York: Simon & Schuster, 1969. $4.95 pb.

Sweetgall, Rob. *Fitness Walking.* Putnam & Sons, 1985. $8.95 pb.

——— and Robert Neeves, Ph.D. *Walking for Little Children.* Creative Walking, Inc., Box 699, Newark, Delaware 19711, 1986. $5 pb.

——— and Robert Neeves, Ph.D. *Walking Wellness Student Workbook.* Newark, Delaware: Creative Walking, Inc., Box 699, Newark Delaware 19711. 1986. $5 pb.

———. *Walking Wellness Teacher's Guide,* Creative Walking, Inc., Box 699, Newark, Delaware 19711. 1986. $13 pb.

——— and John Dignam. *The Walker's Journal.* Creative Walking, Inc., Box, 699, Newark, Delaware, 19711, 1986. $8 pb.

*Walking Magazine.* (National magazine with articles of interest to all walkers) PO Box 56561, Boulder, Colorado 80322-6561. $12 per year.

Wallace, Gordon. *The Valiant Heart.* Ralph Tanner Assoc., 1982. Order directly from author: 102 Aztec Street, Prescott, Arizona 86301. $14.70 hb

Weinstein, Marion and William Finley. *Racewalking.* Steven Greene Press. $9.95 pb.

Winkler, Simon. *Walk, Don't Run.* Windward Publishers, 1981. $4.95 pb.

Yanker, Gary. *The Complete Book of Exercise Walking.* Chicago: Contemporary Books Inc., 1983. $8.95 pb.

## Other Pertinent Books of Interest

Anderson, Bob. *Stretching.* Bolinas, California: Shelter Publishing, 20th printing, 1987. $9.95 pb.

Ardell, Donald. *High Level Wellness.* Emmaus Pennsylvania: Rodale Press Inc., 1978 pb.

Bailey, Covert. *Fit or Fat.* Boston: Houghton Mifflin Co., 1977 pb.

Berland, Theodore. *Rating the Diets.* New York: Beekman House, 1980 hb.

Bland, Jeffrey, Ph.D. *Nutraerobics.* San Francisco: Harper & Row, 1983. $16.95 hb.

Cooper, Kenneth, M.D. *The Aerobics Program for Total Well-Being.* Bantam Books, 1982 pb.

Culligan, Matthew and Keith Sedlacek, M.D. *How to Avoid Stress Before it Kills You.* New York: Gramercy Publishing Co., 1980 hb.

Dufty, William. *Sugar Blues.* Warner Books, 1976 pb.

Galton, Lawrence. *How Long Will I Live?* New York: Macmillan Publishing Co., 1976 hb.

Garrison, Robert and Elizabeth Somer. *The Nutrition Desk Reference.* New Canaan, Connecticut: Keats Publishing Inc., 1985 hb.

Glasser, William, M.D. *Positive Addiction.* New York: Harper & Row, 1976 hb.

Goldbeck, Nikki and David. *The Supermarket Handbook.* New American Library Inc., 1976. pb. (Hardcover by Harper & Row)

Halsell, Grace. *Los Viejos: Secrets of Long Life from the Sacred Valley* Emmaus, Pennsylvania: Rodale Press Inc., 1976 hb.

Hofer, Leonard and Nathan Pritikin. *Live Longer Now.* Grosset and Dunlap, 1974 pb.

Ingils, Brian and Ruth West. *The Alternative Health Guide.* London: Dorling Kindersley Limited, 1983 hb.

Jackson, Ian. *The Breathplay Approach To Whole Life Fitness.* Dolphin/ Doubleday. hb.

Lappé, Frances Moore. *Diet For a Small Planet.* New York: Ballantine Books, 1976 pb.

Lowry, Ron and Ken Sidney. *Orienteering Skills and Strategies.* Orienteering, Ontario: 1220 Sheppard Avenue, E. Willowdale, Ontario, Canada, 1985 pb.

Melleby, Alexander. *The Y's Way to a Healthy Back.* New Century Publishers Inc., 1982 pb.

Pritikin, Nathan. *The Pritikin Program for Diet and Exercise.* Bantam, 1980. pb.

Robertson, Laurel, Carol Flinders and Brownwen Godfrey. *Laurel's Kitchen.* Berkeley, California: Nilgiri Press, 1976. hb.

Segerberg, Osborn, Jr. *Living To Be 100.* New York: Charles Scribner's Sons, 1982. hb.

Seiden, Othniel, M.D. *Coping With Your Bad Back.* Blue Ridge Summit, Pennsylvania: TAB Books Inc., 1984. $6.95 pb.

———. *Coping With Diabetes.* Blue Ridge Summit, Pennsylvania: TAB Books Inc.,1984. $6.95 pb.

———. *Coping with Miscarriage.* Blue Ridge Summit, Pennsylvania: TAB Books Inc., 1984. $6.95 pb.

Selye, Hans, M.D. *The Stress of Life.* McGraw-Hill Book Co., 1978 pb.

Sharkey, Brian. *Physiology of Fitness.* 2nd Edition, Champaign, Illinois: Human Kinetics Publishers, Inc., 1984. $13.95 pb.

Sheehan, George, M.D. *Dr. Sheehan on Fitness.* New York: Simon & Schuster, Inc., 1984 pb.

Traditional Chinese Medicine, (translated to English), *A Barefoot Doctor's Manual.* New York: Gramercy Publishing Co., 1985 hb.

Walford, Roy L., M.D. *Maximum Lifespan* . New York: Avon Books, 1984 pb.

Winter, Ruth. *The Scientific Case Against Smoking.* New York: Crown Publishers Inc., 1980 pb.

Wolfe, Sidney, M.D., and Christopher Coley. *Pills That Don't Work.* New York: Farrar, Straus & Giroux, 1981 pb.

Young, John G., M.D. *S.E.L.E.C.T.: Creative/Innovative Approaches.* Buffalo, New York: Bearly Limited, 1986 pb.

*—Prices when given are as of 1987*

# INDEX

# ABOUT THE AUTHORS

**Bob Carlson** is a veteran of the famed 10th Mountain Division of World War II and a former architect, who gave up his profession in the mid-1970s to devote his life to health promotion and physical fitness. He started as a marathon runner in 1967, but since 1982 has gravitated to walking, especially racewalking, as a far more sensible form of staying in excellent shape. Bob has won many racewalking regional championships and a national one in his 60-64 age group, normally doing the 5 kilometer distance in 29 to 30 minutes. He has done extensive writing and teaching on the benefits of walking as the best exercise for the most people. He is the founder of Colorado's Front Range Walkers Club.

**O.J. Seiden, M.D.,** quit his medical practice in the middle 1970s to become an author writing mostly on health-related subjects. He also volunteers his time periodically to assist an organization called Doctors to the World, which sends physicians to underdeveloped sectors of the earth, to establish better health practices. Dr. Seiden would love to see the entire populace embrace his own lifestyle habits, of which endurance walking is the cornerstone. His best effort is 78 miles—a triple marathon—in about 18 hours.

3

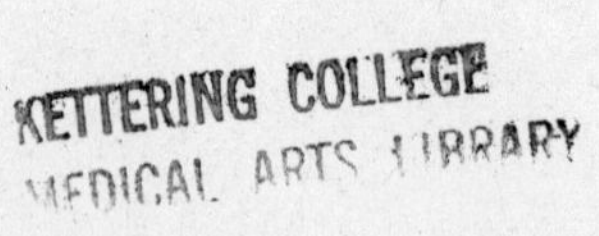